"There's a revolution in healthcare that is being led by medical extended reality. *Virtual Reality for Serious Illness* brings together some of the leading voices who share their experience, insights, and passion for this innovative new field. It's a great resource for medical students and professionals and for the artists and creative technologists who want to help create virtual experiences for patients in need, or as we say, VR for good. The amazing case studies alone will make the readers join the ranks of medical VR evangelists."

Max Almy, *MFA, former dean of creative technology at the Savannah College of Art and Design*

"This book is on the leading edge and is immensely valuable."

Sara Plaspohl, *DrPH, CHES, formerly associate dean of Waters College of Health Professions*

I0025716

Virtual Reality for Serious Illness

Virtual Reality for Serious Illness explores the important role virtual-reality interventions can play in symptom management, anxiety control, and spiritual meaning. This book focuses on cutting-edge research and its effects on the seriously ill and those who treat the seriously ill. The innovation in this book is twofold: It is a global view of the use of virtual reality in complex medical cases where it takes an interdisciplinary look at the use of virtual reality; and it includes a strong focus on the spiritual healing resulting from the meaning and purpose found during this intervention.

This book is written for professionals who use holistic healing measures in the scope of treatment for chronic and seriously ill patients. It is written for all disciplines acting in holistic healthcare healing, including physicians, chaplains, nurses, and informatics interventionists.

Kathleen D. Benton, PhD, MS, is the president and CEO for a Savannah-area hospice and palliative-care organization. Previously, she served as the director of ethics and palliative care at St. Joseph's/Candler Hospital for over a decade.

Teri Yarbrow, MFA, MS, is the president and CEO of MagikaVRx, founder of Creating AWE, a VR evangelist, and professor of immersive medicine at the Mercer University School of Medicine.

Virtual Reality for Serious Illness

Edited by Kathleen D. Benton and Teri Yarbrow

Routledge
Taylor & Francis Group

NEW YORK AND LONDON

Designed cover image: © Radiance VR Image: Created by
Teri Yarbrow, Max Almy, and Josephine Leong

First published 2025
by Routledge
605 Third Avenue, New York, NY 10158

and by Routledge
4 Park Square, Milton Park, Abingdon, Oxon, OX14 4RN

Routledge is an imprint of the Taylor & Francis Group, an informa business

ISBN: 9781032639642 (hbk)
ISBN: 9781032649757 (pbk)
ISBN: 9781032649771 (ebk)

DOI: 10.4324/9781032649771

Typeset in Palatino
by codeMantra

This is dedicated to my mother, Shirlee Yarbrow, whose passing changed my life. In her final days, she longed for spiritual comfort and closure so I used an iPod to play her favorite arias and classical music as she began her inward journey. Her transition had a profound effect on me as I literally watched her spirit leaving her body and realized that so much more could be done for end-of-life. I was inspired years later to take my first VR work to patients in hospice and palliative care and I saw firsthand the transformative power of VR.

—Teri Yarbrow

Always to Daniel—whose paradoxical suffering coupled with life enjoyment forced him to find innovative and progressive tools in care, hence his love for VR as a professional patient of 30 years. And to all of those who support me every day, to take on too many projects. Namely, all the Bentons, all the DeLoaches, the Girl Tribe, and Christine and Erin—a family and peer group supports longevity in life and in projects.

—Kathleen D. Benton

Contents

Contributors

Erin Allen, MPH, is the senior projects coordinator at Hospice Savannah and senior director for a local hospice collaborative network

Franca Benini, MD, serves as the head of the Veneto Regional Reference Center for Pediatric Pain Management and Palliative Care at the Padua University Hospital in Padua, Italy.

Kathleen D. Benton, PhD, MS, is the president and CEO for a Savannah-area hospice and palliative-care organization. Previously, she served as the director of ethics and palliative care at St. Joseph's/Candler Hospital for over a decade. She earned her doctorate in public health leadership from Georgia Southern University, her master's in bioethics from Case Western Reserve University, and her undergraduate degree in political science and communications from Furman University.

Alice Chirico, PhD, is at the Research Center in Communication Psychology (PSICOM), Faculty of Arts and Philosophy, Catholic University of Milan.

Jose Ferrer Costa, MD, is a primary care physician at Badalona Serveis Assistencials in Badalona, Spain. He is also a medical acupuncturist, clinical tutor for residents, and virtual-reality content developer.

Marianna Graziosi, MA, MAPP, is at the Center for Psychedelic and Consciousness Research, Department of Psychiatry and Behavioral Sciences, Johns Hopkins University School of Medicine.

Sarah Hill is a 12-time mid-America Emmy award-winning former TV journalist who developed Healium for herself as well as the millions of others who want to self heal their anxiety for better sleep and human performance. Healium's roots are in virtual travel for veterans. In 2015, Hill's team built a program called Honor Everywhere, which uses virtual reality and augmented reality to allow aging veterans the opportunity to virtually visit their WWII, Vietnam, Korea, and Women's memorials.

Anna Mercante, MD, serves as a doctor of medicine in child neuropsychiatry at the University Hospital of Padua, Italy.

Nidhi A. Patel received her BSPH from UofSC and is an MHA candidate (graduating May 2024) at Georgia Southern University, Armstrong. She is also a graduate assistant for the Jiann-Ping Hsu College of Public Health at Georgia Southern and works at Hospice Savannah as projects team assistant.

Marta Pizzolante, MSc, is at the Research Center in Communication Psychology (PSICOM), Catholic University of Milan.

Brennan Spiegel, MD, MSHS, is a professor of medicine and public health, director of Health Services Research, and director of master's degree program in Health Delivery Science, Cedars-Sinai site director, Clinical and Translational Science Institute in Cedars-Sinai, Los Angeles, California.

David B. Yaden, PhD, is at the Center for Psychedelic and Consciousness Research, Department of Psychiatry and Behavioral Sciences, Johns Hopkins University School of Medicine

Teri Yarbrow, MS, MFA, is the Founder of Creating AWE, President Magika VRx, and Professor of XR Medicine at Mercer University School of Medicine. She is a Founding Member of AMXRA, XR Health Strategist and VR Evangelist. She is an Emmy Award-winning Creative Director, Producer and Immersive Media Artist.

Yee Hui Yeo, MD, MSc, is a clinical fellow in the Karsh Division of Gastroenterology and Hepatology, Department of Medicine, Cedars-Sinai Medical Center. He is also an active investigator in epidemiology, artificial intelligence, and health outcomes research.

Anna Zanin, MD, is a consultant in pediatric palliative care and pain management in the Department of Women and Child for Padua University in Padua, Italy.

Mark Zhang, MD, Palliative Care Physician at Dana-Farber Cancer Institute, serves as Chief Innovation Officer at the VHA Office of Healthcare Innovation. As the founder and president of the American Medical Extended Reality Association, Dr. Zhang pioneered the integration of extended-reality technologies in healthcare.

Foreword

Mark Zhang

The beginnings of medical extended reality (MXR) date back as late as the 1980s and into the 1990s and were originally utilized for simulations and psychotherapy, but technology has evolved considerably since those early efforts. Medicine has grown around technology.[1] I've personally seen how the future is crafted and moved forward by these big leaps. These leaps are what MXR represents. Such technology-based advancements will define what is needed to meet humanity's needs in the future, and we are at the beginning of what could be a huge opportunity. This book and other efforts signal the readiness of this important growth, both in the field of virtual medicine and in the field of palliative care.

Now we are seeing expansion across the area of MXR into pain mitigation, rehabilitation, many psychological interventions (including meditation), and even enhancing skills and surgical fields across medicine. I am proud to be a founder of the American Medical Extended Reality Association, which started in 2022. This society advances MXR as a new specialty within medical training. We're dedicated to the broadening of that field. The mission is to specifically advance the science and practice of medical extended reality, promoting its best practices in the delivery of care, furthering scientific investigation, supporting innovation, and being a part of the advocacy and education.

Furthermore, out of that society came the *Journal of Medical Extended Reality*, a peer-reviewed effort at exploring new science and research in this advancing area. *Virtual Reality for Serious Illness* takes on something even more unique than the beginnings of this broadening field: It is the first of its kind to collaborate efforts on virtual reality for the seriously ill patient. Palliative medicine and the use of extended reality in hospice and palliative medicine are also relatively new, but in fact, the entire field of palliative care has become the fifth-largest subspecialty in the field with great opportunities for growth but not enough resources. MXR has the ability to add resources and tools to the toolbox of the palliative physician and palliative care. *Virtual Reality for Serious Illness* looks at specifics in pain mitigation, psychosocial interventions, and enhancement of the dignity of the patient through the use of MXR. As a constant advocate for the field of immersive therapies, I am encouraged at the works across the globe researching what more can be done to help those who are truly suffering through their progressive illness as well as those who will ultimately die of their terminal illness.

It is an exciting time in healthcare to find that different interventions combined with technological inventions can change the quality of life and the trajectory of disease for the vulnerable patient. It is most important to be reflective of best practices, to be aware of advances in technology, and to consider societal pressures and norms that shift as humans adapt and grow. This book considers the challenges that practitioners and patients face today in healthcare. It considers the short staffing, the caregiver burnout, and the disproportionate populations that must be cared for well. This gives opportunity for MXR to be active and progressive in a relatively new area of healthcare.

Note

1 Zhang, H., & Spiegel, B. (2024). Introducing the journal of medical extended reality. *Journal of Medical Extended Reality*, *1*(1), 1–3. https://doi.org/10.1089/jmxr.2024.28999.editorial

1

Case Studies in Virtual Reality

Kathleen D. Benton and Teri Yarbrow

Virtual reality (VR) in healthcare is a recent addition to research in the use of symptom and pain management, anxiety control, and helping patients find meaning in illness, especially near end of life.[1]

Palliative care is defined by the World Health Organization as "improving the quality of life of patients and their families who are facing challenges associated with life-threatening illness, whether physical, psychological, social, or spiritual." By its very definition, palliative care seeks to treat patients and their families holistically. It improves the quality of life of caregivers as well. VR can be a powerful therapy for working with the seriously ill and their families, transforming the patient experience.

VR is a fully immersive experience that allows users to explore and interact with virtual spaces, achieved through devices such as head-mounted displays or headsets. The use of VR in medical settings has been studied and implemented by a great number of researchers and programs worldwide. Over 19,000 studies and research papers have been published about VR in healthcare so far. VR immersive therapy is successfully used in leading hospitals, health centers, and for in-home care.

Presence is the magic of virtual reality (VR), the feeling that you're actually in the virtual world. Presence will

DOI: 10.4324/9781032649771-1

cause the user to suspend disbelief and believe they are in the virtual environment, reacting to stimuli as if they were in the real world. It's the holy grail, the purpose of VR.[2]

Presence is what creates immersion. Studies show that it takes the brain less than 30 seconds to believe that a simulation is real and enables the user to be physically present in a nonphysical world. It doesn't matter how true to life an experience may be; the brain can be hijacked into accepting the reality of a new virtual synthetic environment. VR shares with the brain the same basic mechanism: embodied simulations.[3]

Embodiment is the VR property that enables a user to inhabit a world. Embodiment enables users to fly, swim, explore, and experience three-dimensional (3D) digital environments and transcend the limitations of their physical body. For the seriously ill, this can be a rare opportunity to escape the confines of their condition. Immersion is powerful for these patients, as it can relieve anxiety, reduce pain, provide relief, provide physical and mental stimulation, and improve quality of life.

Chronic pain is a real and everyday issue for many patients in both hospice and palliative care. As the World Health Organization states, "Pain is one of the most frequent and serious symptoms experienced by patients in need of palliative care."[4] Distraction therapy techniques and other forms of anxiety reduction are used in palliative and hospice care, and these types of treatments are being greatly enhanced with the use of VR therapy.

An early example that proved the effectiveness of VR therapy for pain relief was *SnowWorld*, a fully immersive VR experience designed by Hunter Hoffman and David Patterson at the University of Washington in 1996. *SnowWorld*, developed at the University of Washington's Human Interface Technology Lab in collaboration with the Harborview Burn Center, was the first immersive virtual world designed for reducing pain.[5]

SnowWorld was specifically designed to help burn patients during the change of wound dressings. In VR, patients tossed snowballs at penguins, which proved to be highly effective during the painful procedures. "Burn patients experienced 35 to 50 percent less pain when immersed in VR, about the same reduction as a moderate dose of opioid painkillers."[6]

There is scientific evidence that suggests VR can help distract people from pain.[7] The gate control theory of pain states that the brain puts up a neurological gate to block pain impulses. When the prefrontal cortex is stimulated in problem solving, inter-activity, or a deep immersion, the brain blocks other impulses.[8] The perception of pain is also a factor in distraction therapy. Pain is subjective and also dependent on attention.[9] Being immersed in another world can transport patients during pain episodes, as it causes them to focus on something other than their pain and or anxiety. In addition, VR has proven to be an excellent vehicle to induce experiences of awe. Researchers have found that awe can stimulate the brain to release oxytocin and endorphins, thus blocking pain.

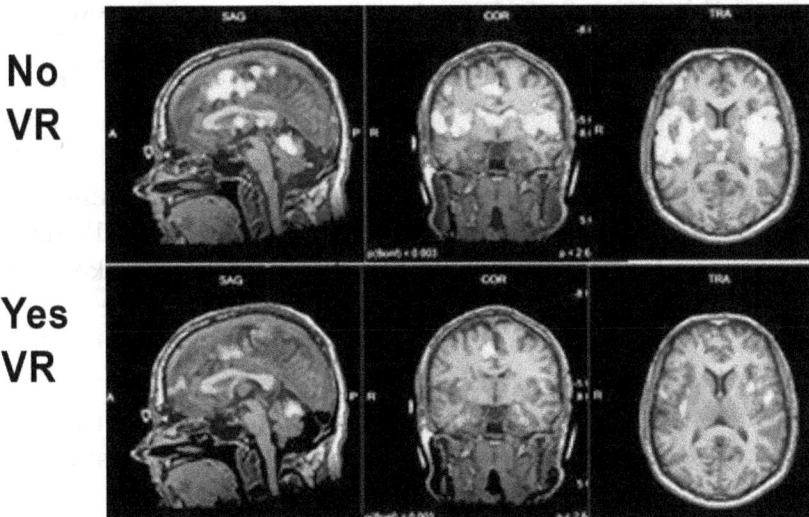

FIGURE 1.1 Pain research using fMRI brain scans show significant reductions in pain-related brain activity during *SnowWorld* in healthy volunteers getting thermal pain stimulations. Image credit Todd Richards and Aric Bills, copyright Hunter Hoffman, vrpain.com.

Why VR for the Seriously Ill

Recent data from the Centers for Disease Control (CDC) show that more than 20% of Americans suffer from chronic pain, and 36% of those have high-impact chronic pain.[10] Approximately 56.8 million people need palliative care each year, including 25.7 million during their end of life.[11] About 70%–90% of the patients experience pain in at least one moment during the palliative phase.[12] Opioids are a standard medication for pain management at the end of life.[13]

In April 2021, Benton, Yarbrow, Gaule, and Perdue launched an Institutional Review Board (IRB)-approved study on the effects of VR on pain and anxiety for palliative-care patients being seen in the Steward Center for Palliative Care's outpatient clinic. The purpose of this VR study was to test and monitor the short-term and long-term effectiveness of virtual-reality therapy with palliative-care patients with progressing illnesses. The data collected was focused on understanding the relief of pain, depression, anxiety, and opioid dependence using VR and tracked the effects of these sessions over an eight- to ten-week period.

Participants

The participants eligible for this therapy were home-based palliative-care patients and palliative-care patients in the Nancy N. and J. C. Lewis Cancer and Research Pavilion clinic under the care of Hospice Savannah and the Steward Center for Palliative Care. The chosen participants had the abilities to make cognitive decisions and were ages 18-plus or under 18 with parental consent. The VR therapy sessions were conducted in 20- to 30-minute increments, weekly. The participants were asked to fill out presession surveys and postsession surveys on a Likert scale of 1–10 to determine their pain levels, the type(s) of pain they were feeling, location of the pain, and whether they were experiencing any anxiety.

Figure 1.2 shows the survey used in this research.

The chance of risk for participating in this study was low to minimal; however, it was possible that a participant might experience anxiety from the immersive nature of VR in

Pre-Participation Pain Assessment Survey:

1. On a scale of 1-10, what is your level of pain?

1	2	3	4	5	6	7	8	9	10

2. Would you describe your pain as constant or intermittent?

Constant	Intermittent

3. Are there any alleviating or aggravating factors for your pain?

4. Could you indicate where you feel pain?

5. What words would you use to describe your pain?

6. Are you currently experiencing anxiety due to your pain?

Post-Participation Pain Assessment Survey:

1. On a scale of 1-10, what is your level of pain?

1	2	3	4	5	6	7	8	9	10

2. Are you currently experiencing any anxiety?

3. Do you feel your participation in the Virtual Reality Program provided you with any relief?

   a) Circle YES or NO

4. Do you feel that you would benefit from additional experiences within this program?

   a) Circle YES or NO

FIGURE 1.2

addition to nausea or dizziness from perceived motion. The foreseeable benefits associated with participating in this study were alleviation of pain without the use of narcotics. There was also anticipation of seeing a decrease in palliative-care patients' anxiety levels. These benefits expand beyond the participants in this study to the general population as well. Through the participation of these terminally ill patients and those with chronic pain, the researchers gathered data on how to use technology to provide alternative forms of symptom management rather than relying solely on narcotics and prescription pain medicine. It was hoped that the virtual-reality therapy sessions would result in a reduction of at least 25% of the pain in enrolled subjects.

Results

Approximately 84.62% of the participants in our study expressed improvement in their pain levels; 61.54% of participants experienced 50% improvement in their pain levels immediately after the VR experience; and 23.1% of participants experienced more than 50% improvement. All 100% of the participants expressed that they benefited from receiving the single VR experience, and 96.2% expressed that additional VR experiences were beneficial to them.

What this study shows is the effectiveness in palliative care for pain reduction and anxiety relief. The first-of-its-kind study

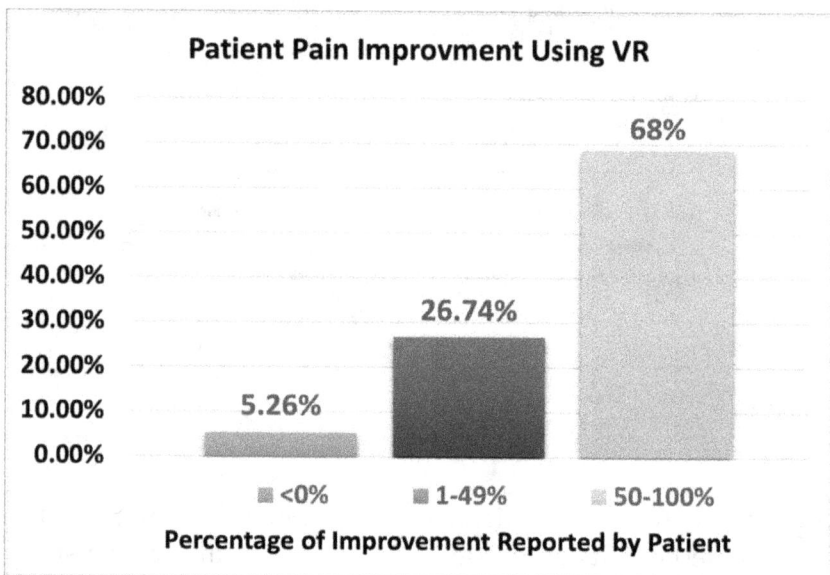

FIGURE 1.3 STATs × Patients Across Palliative.

results are very encouraging in a population that suffers from terminal illness.

Case Studies

The following are a few of the case studies from working in palliative care and hospice that illustrate how beneficial VR can be in the lives of patients.

Louisa: Wonder and Awe

Louisa was a patient with stage IV pancreatic cancer and she had a bucket-list request to go skydiving. As a hospice homecare patient, she was obviously too weak to skydive but VR could bring the experience to her. Finding soothing skydiving 360-degree experiences was quite challenging as there were many with rock and heavy metal music accompanying the visuals. The objective was to provide an exhilarating immersive experience without creating terrifying, heightened anxiety or motion sickness.

Louisa's first experience with VR enabled her to skydive over Rio de Janeiro to the music of Beethoven. Next, she soared through clouds over the Dolomite mountains in Italy and down ski slopes. It was enlivening for her to experience the freedom of flying untethered through the sky through the power of immersive technology. Eleanor Roosevelt once said, "Do one thing every day that scares you." Skydiving is a powerful metaphor for letting go and for the release that Louisa desired in her diminished state.

After she experienced *Wingsuit over Yosemite*, her session concluded with a more meditative experience, *Radiance VR*. The tension visibly left Louisa's body and she commented, "Wow, that's so beautiful, so cool!... Amazing!" VR brought wonder and awe to a patient confined to homecare and daytime television. This was the first VR immersive therapy session conducted in the program and the start of the partnership with VR, hospice, and palliative care.

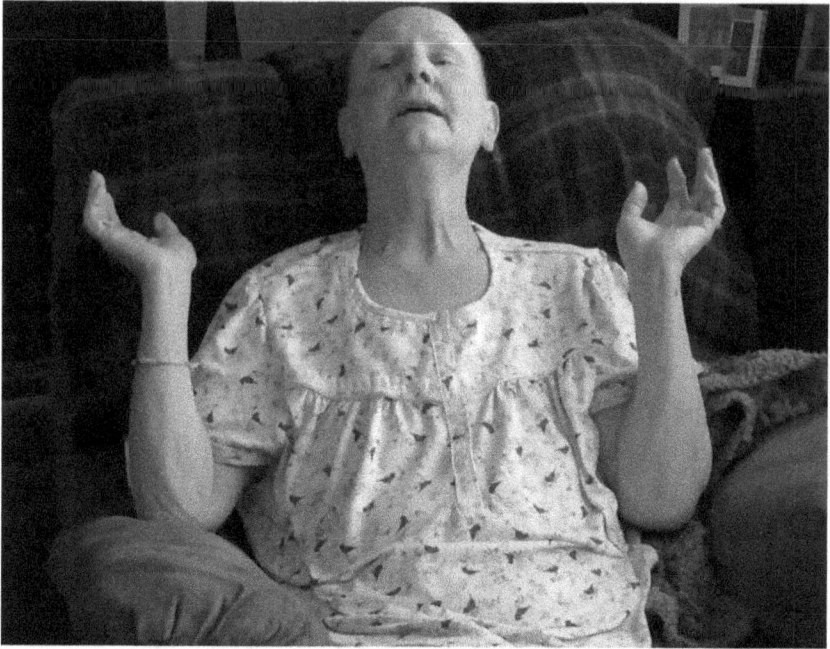

FIGURE 1.4 Louisa after experiencing VR.

Joan: VR for Pain Management

Joan was a 62-year-old woman who became quadriplegic from a car accident in 2019. In addition to paralysis, she had severe neuropathic pain from her shoulders through her arms and hands. To keep Joan comfortable, she was prescribed pain medication, which did little to alleviate her painful condition. Her sleep was affected as well, and she had night terrors. She began VR sessions twice a week for an hour in the summer of 2020.

Joan was in a pain episode and didn't want to be touched. Her bed was adjusted so she was partially upright and gently fitted with an Oculus Quest headset. Her session began with dolphin play, a meditative underwater live-action experience with soothing music. It's an immersive experience where one feels surrounded by a huge pod of dolphins swimming directly in front, above, below, and behind. The soundscape is atmospheric music with dolphin sounds of clicks, chirps, squeals, and whistles. All of this contributes to the sensation of "presence."

Joan loved the dolphin experience so much that she repeated it four continuous times. She laughed and smiled, said she was beginning to feel better and was ready for more VR. This was the beginning of the work to find immersive experiences to transport Joan from her awareness of physical pain and her incapacitating condition to engaging experiences that were fulfilling and improved her quality of life.

During that summer, Joan traveled virtually to Paris, Venice, and the Great Wall of China and experienced the Northern Lights, to name just a few, through a Savannah College of Art and Design (SCAD) student VR project called Born to Roam. This VR experience is part of the VR for Good Project and is a hot-air balloon adventure that starts locally and takes the viewer on the trip of a lifetime. Joan expressed that what she really liked was the feeling of moving on a gondola in Venice. For someone who cannot move, VR can provide a sense of agency, the ability to have a little control over their environment. For Joan, it was a powerful release. Finding experiences with action, motion, and flight became a theme for her sessions. She experienced flying with butterfly migrations, gliding over waterfalls, swimming, snorkeling, sailing, kayaking in Hawaii, and many more.

Joan also loved *Nalu, Heart of the Ocean*, another experience from SCAD's VR for Good Project. This 11-minute, deeply immersive experience transports the viewer to an idyllic coral reef. The viewer observes the slow changes over the course of a day and night, as dolphins, jellyfish, schools of coral fish, and a whale pass by. The soundscape is hauntingly beautiful, filled with underwater sounds. Joan remarked after experiencing *Nalu*: "It made me feel very relaxed… It diminished my pain… It was truly amazing… I still have no pain." This is an example of the gate theory, which suggests that when the prefrontal cortex is stimulated in deep immersion, a neurological gate blocks the pain.[14]

Her sessions always began with the dolphin experience to help relieve the pain and anxiety. A Wong-Baker pain-rating scale with facial expressions was used to measure Joan's pain at the beginning of her sessions and at the end. Joan's husband, Clark, her primary caregiver, kept track of how long the effect of no pain lasted. Often Joan's pain began at 8 and dropped to 0 pain and would last six to eight hours. Clark stated, "It's a miracle... Joan is sleeping better, and I can finally get some sleep!"

Numerous studies have tracked the lasting effects of VR therapy beyond the patient sessions. As in this case study, VR proved extremely effective, providing relief from anxiety and pain. A study of the impact of VR on neuropathic pain in 2018 found that with acute pain,

> the VR sessions provided significant pain relief in all treatment sessions with an average of a 66% reduction in pain during the VR session and a 45% reduction in pain immediately after the session. A decrease in pain was reported to last an average of *30 hours after the session*.[15]

Joan's positive response to VR led her deeper into immersive therapy. She was searching for answers to help explain the reason for her accident and her untreatable condition and she hoped for a home visit from her pastor. So many chaplains, ministers, and rabbis are spread very thin, so Joan had to weather her "dark night of the soul" alone. Although she enjoyed travel experiences, as the reality of her physical condition and its constraints sunk in, she expressed that she wanted more experiences that were profound. *Conscious Existence: A Journey Within* resonated with her. "You are gifted every moment with life's most precious achievement: a conscious mind, enabling you to sense and hold within, the universe's boundless beauty—a source of infinite inspiration that fuels your inner space."[16]

Joan watched *Conscious Existence* and *Radiance VR* multiple times. VR was a powerful tool for Joan to explore spiritual themes in her later sessions so the inner journey through immersive guided meditations was a great liberator for her. Awe induced by VR helped Joan rise above the imprisonment of her body and have self-transcendent experiences (STEs). An STE "allows for the highest levels of unity and harmony within oneself and with the world."[17]

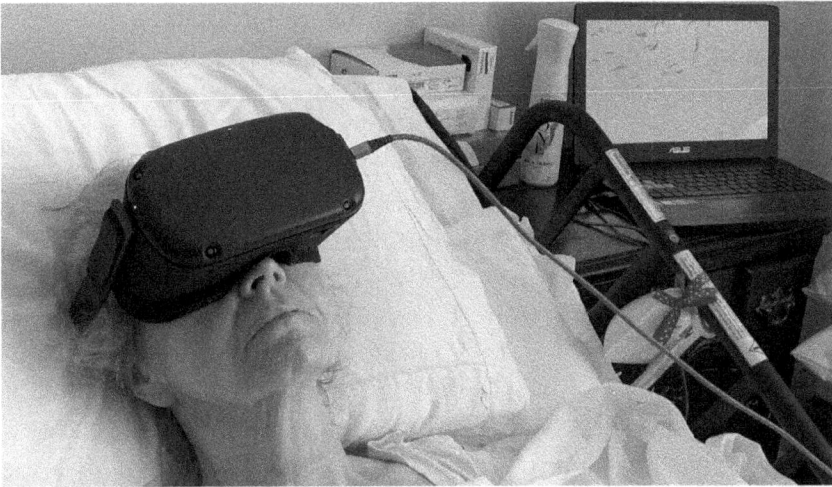

FIGURE 1.5 Joan experiencing *Nalu* in VR.

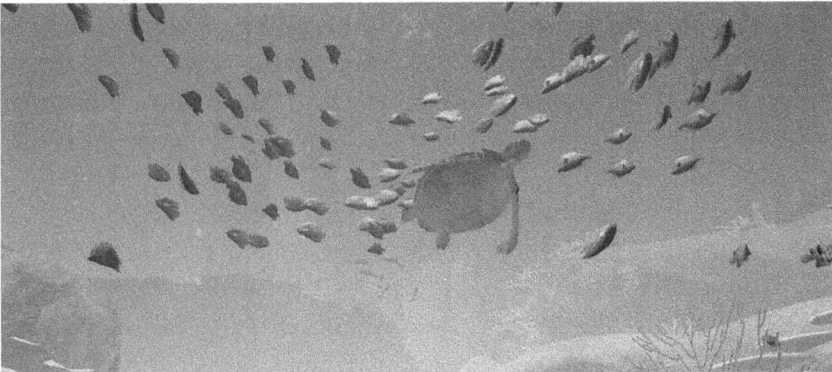

FIGURE 1.6 *Nalu—Heart of the Ocean*, created by Yasmin Alansari, Dante Cameron, Nadav Ben Haim, Katie Howarth, Chanapa ("Gift") Kerdiapee, Maya Peleg, and Conner Witte.

Roger: Restoring a Love of Flight

Roger, a hospice patient on respite care, requested to experience VR. When asked at the beginning of his session if he wanted to go any place in the world, he laughed and said he'd already seen everything! He then asked if there were any plane simulations in VR.

After finding an immersive flight simulation, he was informed that he could experience motion sickness. Once putting on the headset, he completely lit up and began explaining all the mechanics of the inside of the plane. He kept going on and on about how accurate the plane's cockpit was. He got so vocal about it that the session had to move to a different room because the other patient in the next bed wanted some quiet time. On the way over to the other room, he said how amazed he was with VR, even though he had only been in for an initial ten minutes.

Before experiencing another simulation, he shared that for his entire life he had been a pilot and only recently retired. He'd always loved flying and worked with planes in every way—the military, private, commercial, teaching, and so on. He was so fascinated with VR, he asked if he could see a specific plane's interior. The moment he entered the interior, he was overjoyed and said how realistic it was.

Next, he wanted to experience the point of view from the cockpit when the plane is doing tricks. As the simulation began, he verbalized the entire process. He told his audience each of the tricks the plane was doing and talked as if he were over the intercom in the plane.

Roger revealed that he was forced to retire because he was going blind. He then took off the headset and there were tears in his eyes. He was so happy that in VR he could see clearly. He exclaimed, "That made my day and it really felt like I was back on a plane. I could see again! I wish I could have gotten introduced to VR sooner!"

Betty: Memory Care

Betty was in memory care, depressed, and in chronic pain. She often stayed in bed most of the day without remembering anything about herself. She believed she was going to die soon, so had no reason to get out of bed. Formerly a happily married woman who was cultured and well-traveled, Betty's world had grown very insular within her apartment in assisted living and the effects of dementia. With great coaxing to get her out of bed and making sure her hearing aids were in place, she began virtual-reality sessions. She traveled in VR to Venice, Paris, Amsterdam, and Vienna. Her first immersive experiences reminded her of her travels with her deceased husband. Her mood improved and she was willing to get dressed for dinner.

Over the next few visits, she began to experience the arts in VR: the Paris Ballet, visits to the Louvre, traveling inside Monet paintings, visiting Van Gogh's immersive Starry Night, a dance performance from *West Side Story*, behind the scenes of the Australian Ballet, and many more.

As a young child, her family took her to the symphony, and she grew up playing classical music on the piano. Betty's attitude improved and she would get up for her VR sessions with immersive classical music. She experienced Ravel's *Bolero* numerous times, Beethoven's *Fifth*, Beethoven's *Ninth*, Grieg's *Peer Gynt Suite*, Vivaldi's *Four Seasons*, Tchaikovsky piano concertos, Brahms, among others. She sat in rapture and moved her hands as if she were conducting, humming along with this great music.

Music therapy has long been used as an effective therapy to calm anxiety, relieve depression, and improve quality of life for patients with all types of distress and illness. In addition, music has been found to be very effective at triggering memory.

> Listening to and performing music reactivates areas of the brain associated with memory, reasoning, speech, emotion, and reward. Two recent studies—one in the United States and the other in Japan—found that music doesn't just help us retrieve stored memories, it also helps us lay down new ones.[18]

In addition, "Music is found to be one of the common elicitors of awe."[19] Awe-inspiring music combined with compelling visuals and the visceral immersive effects of VR can create a strongly positive benefit for a patient's mental and physical well-being.

The most profound result of Betty's VR sessions was the day when, after watching Beethoven's *Ode to Joy* in VR, she walked over to her piano and played it from memory!

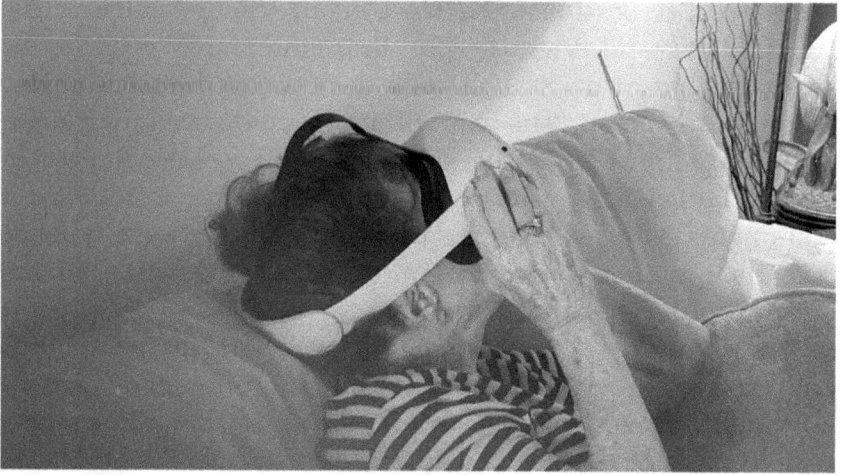

FIGURE 1.7 Betty experiencing VR.

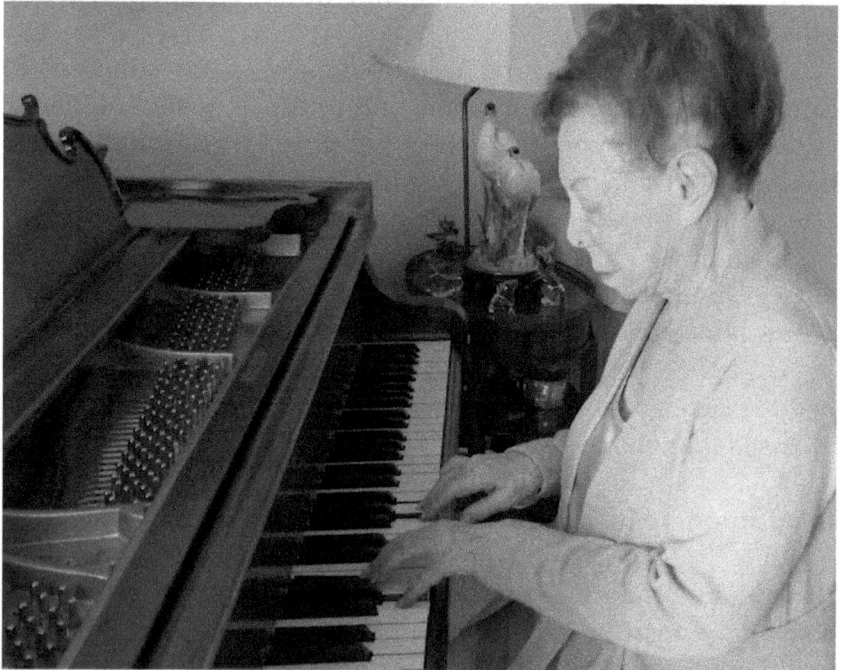

FIGURE 1.8 Betty playing *Ode to Joy* after her VR session.

Debbie: Journey from Isolation

A 52-year-old patient struggling with ovarian cancer at the palliative-care clinic, Debbie's treatment had led to extreme weight gain, hair loss, and skin issues. Her husband was extremely unsupportive and had isolated himself from the illness journey. He would not accompany Debbie to any doctor's appointments. He even had gone so far as to insult her physical appearance, jokingly asking her to pursue diet pills at the doctor's visit. Debbie had no other family and felt isolated at work, especially as her productivity had waned due to ongoing symptoms. She was experiencing suicidal ideations and in fact called her oncologist to express her concern for her own depression. She called the oncology office one weekend again expressing the suicidal concerns. Her oncologist sent her to palliative care for full support.

She was greeted by the VR therapist and was immediately calmed by the program. She began to cry at the onset of the VR experience. She reported that it was the first time she had felt any joy or hope during the duration of her illness. Before even being seen by the doctor for symptom control, she reported feeling lighter and finally smiled once again. She went on to explain to the VR therapist how hopeless she had felt and how this experience reminded her that there is a bigger world outside her disease, outside the lack of support she received in her own life. It inspired her to connect with group support and to even plan a trip that she had convinced herself she would not be able to make. Sometime later, she made the trip to Hawaii.

Sam: Enhancing Quality of Life

Sam, a former high school science teacher, had amyotrophic lateral sclerosis (ALS). He had been confined to his chair for more than five years. With the loss of mobility and motor coordination, VR offered a release from the limitations of Sam's condition. Finding the correct fit for the headset was the first task, as his neck couldn't support his head and oftentimes he leaned far enough over to turn off the Quest. A long, continuous list of experiences was planned because once the Oculus was seated properly, taking the headset off and on was not easy.

Finding experiences with action, extreme motion, and flight was an ongoing theme for Sam's sessions. He enjoyed hang-gliding, soaring in a wing suit, diving with sharks, and experiences with interstellar content such as exploring the space station, experiencing zero gravity, walking in space, and viewing Earth and the other planets from a different point of view. VR was a release and the high point of his day.

His sessions ended with experiences that had interactive tasks, and one of his favorites was *FlowBorne*, a breathing meditation.

> *FlowBorne* VR was created by psychologists to provide an intuitive and playful way of learning evidence-based breathing techniques for meditation, relaxation, stress reduction, concentration, and sleep. *FlowBorne* VR was empirically investigated in a peer-reviewed controlled laboratory study. Over the course of just six brief sessions, participants significantly improved their breathing skills and mental health.[20]

The hand controller must be placed on the viewer's stomach to measure breath. This enabled transport in the experience via breath. With a deep breath, Sam moved easily through computer-generated gardens, forests, rivers, and many terrains. With shallower breaths, the movement slows. It was an experience that gave him a sense of "agency" in his world. "Agency in VR refers to the sense of control a user has over their current environment or situation. The higher the agency you give a VR user, the more they should be able to influence the world around them."[21]

Sam lived in a high-end motorized chair so having a sense of agency was a time of freedom and liberation from his condition. Another experience that gave Sam a sense of agency in VR was *Lampsi*. Created by SCAD students in the VR for Good project, *Lampsi* was a gaze-based experience. Most VR is controlled by hand tracking with both hands. Unable to use his hands, *Lampsi* was designed by students when they heard about Sam's

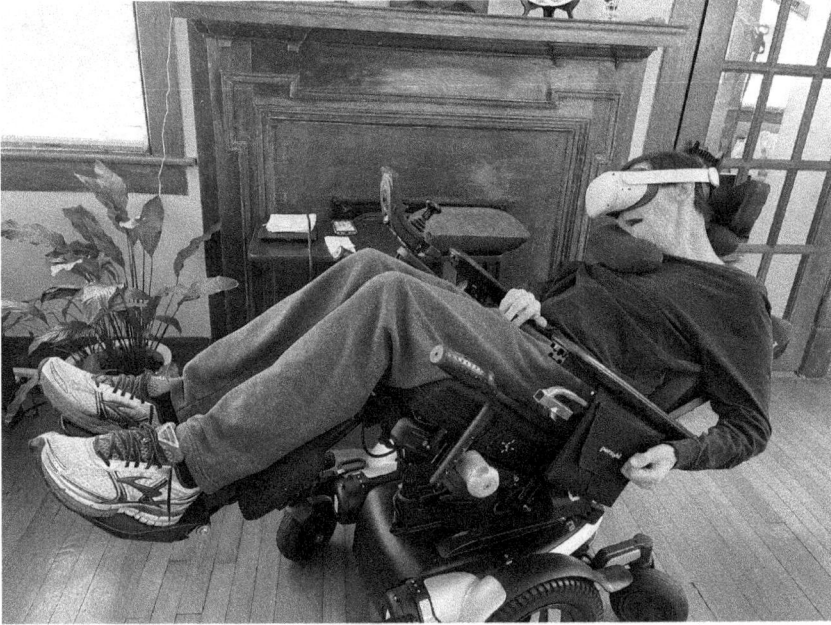

FIGURE 1.9 Sam experiencing VR from his motorized wheelchair.

challenges in VR. They created an experience that was interactive by using one's eyes.

The experience begins in a bioluminescent cave where one is seated in a gondola on a reflective underground river. The viewer stares at a butterfly to initiate movement through the cave utilizing eye-tracking. The journey concludes at sunset on a beach filled with sky lanterns. The music is an atmospheric soundscape with a soothing voice prompting one to engage:

> This is the sea of lanterns, each and every one was released by someone who came before you. Each lantern holds a moment, a memory, celebrated and released into the sky. Take a moment to reflect on a person, place, or experience that you love. Whenever you are ready to release your lantern, look at it to send it on its way…. As your lantern ascends into the sky, notice how you feel…. Take a moment to reflect…. Breathe in and out with the waves and let them wash away your cares.[22]

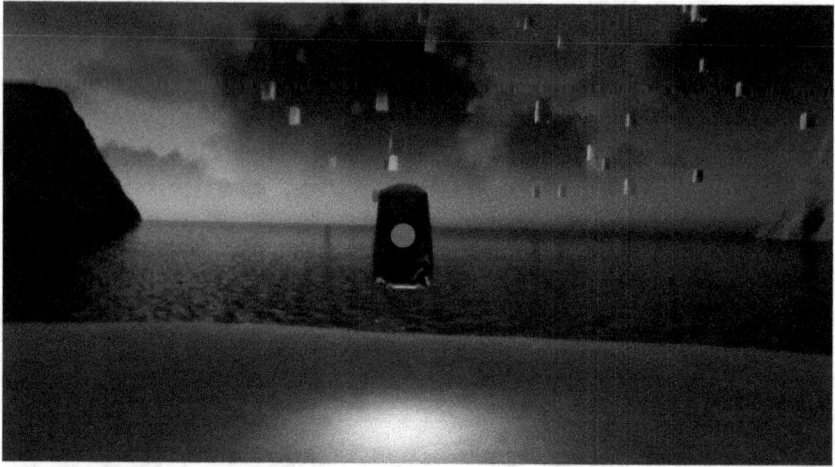

FIGURE 1.10 *The Sea of Lanterns* from *Lampsi VR*, created by Jacob Alexander, Cate Boddy, Jesse Fazzini, Rylee Fisher, Kushal Nataraja Savitha, and Christian Wheeler, 2022.

With the help of his wife, Sam was able to use his eyes to release a sky lantern.

Amyotrophic lateral sclerosis (ALS) is a progressive neurodegenerative disease and currently there is no cure. As Sam's case study clearly shows, VR can enhance the quality of life, sense of well-being, and mental health for many patients. Each case study in this chapter has shown the numerous benefits of VR therapy, from relief of pain, anxiety, and depression to mental acuity and spiritual comfort. One thing remains abundantly clear: this new technology is vital and greatly beneficial for successful care and measurable positive outcomes with seriously ill patients.

References

1 Benton, K., Yarbrow, T., Gaule, M., & Foran, M. (2022). Transforming the palliative care experience with virtual reality. *International Journal of Nursing Health Care Research, 5*, 1340. https://doi.org/10.29011/2688-9501.101340

2   Rogers, S. (2020, March 5). Why XR in the classroom? *VRfocus*. Retrieved from https://www.vortals.app/post/why-xr-in-the-classroom

3   Riva, G., Wiederhold, B., & Matovani, F. (2019, January 1). *Neuroscience of virtual reality: From virtual exposure to embodied medicine*. Retrieved from https://www.ncbi.nlm.nih.gov/pmc/articles/PMC6354552/

4   World Health Organization. (2020, August 5). Palliative care. Retrieved from https://www.who.int/news-room/fact-sheets/detail/palliative-care

5   HITLab, University of Washington. (2008, June 23). Virtual reality pain reduction. Retrieved from http://www.hitl.washington.edu/projects/vrpain/

6   Kenney, T. (2018, February 24). SnowWorld melts away pain for burn patients, using virtual reality snowballs. *Geekwire*. Retrieved from https://www.geekwire.com/2018/snowworld-melts-away-pain-burn-patients-using-virtual-reality-snowballs/#:~:text=It%20might%20seem%20silly%2C%20but,noise%2C'%E2%80%9D%20Hoffman%20said

7   Dauchot, N. (2018, June 1). VR for pain distraction. *Medium*. Retrieved from https://medium.com/uxxr/vr-for-pain-distraction-939b7a5b912d

8   Melzack, R., & Wall, P.D. (1965, November 19). Pain mechanisms: A new theory. *Science*. Retrieved from https://www.science.org/doi/abs/10.1126/science.150.3699.971

9   Ambron, R.T., & Sinav, A. (2022). *The brain and pain: Breakthroughs in neuroscience*. New York: Columbia University Press, 2022.

10 Adams, K. (2022, September). Why VR could be the new dawn of pain. *Anxiety Management*. https://medcitynews.com/2022/09/why-

11 World Health Organization. (2020, August 5). Palliative care. Retrieved from https://www.who.int/news-room/fact-sheets/detail/palliative-care

12 Sholjakova, M., Durnev, V., Kartalov, A., & Kuzmanovska, B. (2018). Pain relief as an integral part of the palliative care. *Open Access Macedonian Journal of Medical Sciences*, 6(4), 739–741. https://doi.org/10.3889/oamjms.2018.163

13 Sinha, M.S., & Dineen Gillespie, K. (2022). Realigning incentives for novel pain therapeutics. *Anesthesiology, 137*, 134–136. https://doi.org/10.1097/ALN.0000000000004287

14 Melzack, R., & Wall, P.D. (1965, November 19). Pain mechanisms: A new theory. *Science.* Retrieved from https://www.science.org/doi/abs/10.1126/science.150.3699.971

15 Jones, T., Skadberg, R., & Moore, T. (2018, January 1). A pilot study of the impact of repeated sessions of virtual reality on chronic neuropathic pain. *International Journal of Virtual Reality.* Retrieved from https://ijvr.eu/article/view/2901

16 Harvey, J. (2020, May 26). Conscious existence. An interview with Marc Zimmerman. *LinkedIn.* Retrieved from https://www.linkedin.com/pulse/conscious-existence-interview-marc-zimmermann-john-harvey/

17 Kaufman, S.B. (2020). *Transcend: The new science of self-actualization.* New York: TarcherPerigee.

18 Fabiny, A. (2015, February 14). Music can boost memory and mood. *Harvard Women's Health Watch.* Retrieved from https://www.health.harvard.edu/mind-and-mood/music-can-boost-memory-and-mood#:~:text=Listening%20to%20and%20performing%20music%20reactivates%20areas%20of,it%20also%20helps%20us%20lay%20down%20new%20ones

19 Keltner, D., & Haidt, J. (2003). Approaching awe, a moral, spiritual, and aesthetic emotion. *Cognition & Emotion, 17*(2), 297–314. https://doi.org/10.1080/02699930302297

20 Rockstroh, C., Blum, J., & Göritz, A.S. (2020, October 5). A mobile VR-based respiratory biofeedback game to foster diaphragmatic breathing. *Virtual Reality, 25,* 539–552. https://doi.org/10.1007/s10055-020-00471-5

21 Carter, R. (2021, May 14). Presence or agency: What's the key to virtual engagement? *XR Today.* Retrieved from https://www.xrtoday.com/virtual-reality/presence-or-agency-whats-the-key-to-virtual-engagement/#:~:text=%E2%80%9CAgency%E2%80%9D%20in%20VR%20refers%20to,influence%20the%20world%20around%20them

22 VR for Good team. (2022). *Lampsi VR.* Retrieved from https://about.meta.com/community/vr-for-good/

2

Disconnect between Humanity and Medicine

Kathleen D. Benton, Nidhi A. Patel, and Erin Allen

Healthcare globally has become disjointed, representing a systemic failure in need of disruption. Treatments are protocol driven, and patients are described by their disease—"the ALS in room 415" or "the broken leg in the waiting room"—as if that were the only important facet of their lives. The human condition has been partially left out of what it means to heal; symptoms are sometimes addressed as if one symptom has no bearing on other symptoms. Providers oftentimes document instead of listen. The number of patients takes priority over the care of the patients.

When a terminally ill patient is faced with existential questions, there are no clear-cut answers or concrete evidence of what is to come after death. To attempt to gain clarity on these topics, cultural backgrounds and personal belief systems play an enormous role in this journey for the individual. Aligning the treatment measures to the patient's values and beliefs can cause the patient to find clarity of their belonging to family or group and reduce their feeling of isolation.

DOI: 10.4324/9781032649771-2

The Current State of Healthcare in the United States

The United States has a higher death rate for preventable conditions when compared to many other populations. In fact, the United States ranks in the bottom third of life expectancy. In 2020, the life expectancy in the US was 77 years compared to the Organization for Economic Co-operation and Development (OECD) average of 80.

Further, life expectancy in the United States is expected to continue to decline. The United States has one of the highest preventable mortality rates and, when compared to their peers, the US has a lower rate of physician visits. Many of these statistics are thought to be related to the significant costs of healthcare throughout the country. When compared to similar populations, the cost of healthcare in the United States is significantly higher.

Innovations in healthcare are extremely important. While we cannot change the high costs of healthcare, technology and artificial intelligence (AI) software can provide solutions that can be more readily available, less time consuming, and more cost effective.[1]

Nationally, spending in healthcare exceeds 40% of the US gross national product (GNP). Americans spend more per capita on healthcare than any other country, yet Americans are dissatisfied with their care and are one of the few countries with no national healthcare program. Access to healthcare in the United States is defined by those who can pay. With competition in both the private and public networks, there are layers of barriers.

Public Network

The US government plays a hefty role in dispensing healthcare funds as well as setting regulation for such, but many of the benefits are outdated when practitioners in healthcare are not intertwined to changing or improving regulations to bring them into our modern environment. One example is the hospice benefit. Hospice takes care of patients with terminal illness. The current benefit requires certification by the physician of a six-month prognosis—the patient is not expected to live longer than six months. However, it also allows the physician authority to recertify if the patient lives longer. Currently third-party vendors work diligently to audit and recoup monies where patients live longer under this service, even though the patient remains terminal. Under this same benefit, a patient is only appropriate for inpatient hospice care if they have uncontrolled symptoms. "Uncontrolled symptoms" do not include dying but instead refer to unaddressed pain or agitation. This leads to many hospice patients with no appropriate caregiver and with very little option on where they can die. Another factor is that these two examples of regulatory statutes lead to hospice providers having to pour more resources into compliance staff than they used to, which then results in less care for the complicated dying patient.

Private Network

The US private network is monopolized by insurers that play an avoidance game.[2] For example, if a line is not signed or a specific language not placed in the narrative, they will not pay for comprehensive care. This leads providers to play their own game of high volume and huge efficiencies just to survive financially. This does not allow for human care or compassion, innovation or listening. Put simply, the system works against promotion of holistic care and its full focus on the human condition.

The US healthcare system is one of the largest and fastest growing industries and yet there is great dissatisfaction with care, and the cost of healthcare continues to rise. There are several reasons why this is occurring. The US healthcare industry has a unique characteristic in perceiving healthcare as a right, not a privilege. However, the demand is based on one's ability to pay and yet the providers, rather than the consumers, determine the extent of demand receiving the care.[3] Another concern surrounds the payment methods of Medicare, Medicaid, and private insurances coverage. The implementation of the Medicare/Medicaid Act in 1966 contributed to the rapid rise in healthcare costs.[4] Private insurances have led to inadequate access to care as there are certain limitations on coverage based on the individual's care plan package.[5]

Global Growth Repercussions of an Aging Population

By 2034, retired persons in the United States will outnumber those in schools for the first time in history. America is not alone in facing a hefty aging population. Japan was the first to weather the repercussions.[6] Some of the problems that Japan faced included closing schools; increasing rest breaks to satisfy a labor force of 70–80-year-old employees; and adjustments to labor sites to allow aged personnel with vision and mobility issues to accomplish their work. In addition, accidents involving older employees (60 and older) totaled about 38,000 in Japan in 2022, up 26% from five years earlier. A safe working environment is essential for continued productivity.

In 2050, 80% of the global population is estimated to be in low- and middle-income countries. Our pace of aging is going faster than our growth. In 2020 the number of people aged 60 years and older outnumbered the youth below age 5 for the first time. By 2030, one person in six will be over 60, or approximately 1.4 billion people. This older population will double by 2050, from 12% to 22%.[7] This rise is coupled with a decrease in reproduction and decrease in those going to school to learn how to care for older adults. Thus, between the imbalance of the old and young combined with reduction in healthcare workers coming out of the pandemic emergency years, a perfect storm is born. This perfect storm has no end in sight and innovation is quite literally the only way out. More technological solutions that can be created and accepted for intervention and tools to support and assist caregivers will better the potential for positive outcome in the population of imbalance. There is a pace that has been ignored for years and is only now coming into point of focus, discussion, and solution because of the grave potential for negative healthcare implosion if it is not taken seriously.

The growth in aging in the US is more tangibly seen in travel growth in retirees and packed waiting rooms. Appointments with specialists are not easily achieved and, in some cases, can take months, allowing a minor issue to become more severe. Waiting for healthcare, even in urgent situations, has become a trend. As the aged increase, so too will their ailments. The older we get, the more our comorbidities will increase, thus increasing our need for additional healthcare at a time when it is harder to get.

The overall US healthcare system has a narrow focus on treating the diagnoses rather than the patient as a whole being, with the possible exception of some good end-of-life care. End-of-life care is unique due to its aim to provide a holistic approach of care that comprehensively addresses the well-being of individual by attempting to meet physical and emotional needs as well as psychological and spiritual needs. Because of the earlier shortcomings in patients' illness journeys, a detrimental challenge is created as patients face the uncertainty of what is to come and attempt to find the answers to existential questions in a short amount of time, while also dealing with the neuropathic pain of their illness.

Cultural Implications of End-of-Life Care

Many, if not all, seriously ill patients experience some level of psychogenic pain as they search for answers to existential question like "Why me?" or "Why now?"[8] They long to find meaning and purpose in their lives and a sense of belonging before facing death. A fundamental aspect of human cognition is the innate curiosity that allows them to explain or solve various phenomena throughout their lives. However, when one is faced with existential questions, there are no clear-cut answers or concrete evidence of what is to come after death. To attempt to gain clarity on these topics, cultural backgrounds and personal belief systems play an enormous role in this journey for the individual. Spiritual healing and emotional support can provide patients with a sense of hope and inner peace that, in turn, results in resilience and better coping abilities.[9] However, it is crucial for clinicians to understand a patient's cultural background and personal beliefs to effectively provide culturally competent care.

Culture is frequently misunderstood as a surface-level collection of shared elements like food, music, and clothing choices. However, it is much more than that. Understanding a culture provides an insight into the various complexities of one's life experiences, such as values and beliefs, social norms and customs, history and tradition, and religion and spirituality.[10] All of these elements guide an individual to understanding their belonging and purpose within the context of society, and affect how the individual chooses to navigate the way of life *and* death. It shapes the way an individual views suffering, illness, and death.

Therefore, culture shapes the way individuals approach the fundamental aspects of life and death, providing a lens through which to view and attempt to answer existential questions with ease rather than fear. Each culture and individual within that culture has a unique way of coping with psychogenic pain and with understanding existential phenomenon. For example, Christians often turn to prayer and confession to gain a sense of peace, Buddhists may turn to meditation and mindfulness practices to relieve the nature of suffering and explore existence, Hindus may turn to *antyesti* practices through a series of rituals and ceremonies to guide the soul to its next journey, and atheists may find their purpose through humanistic and philosophical perspectives.

Traditional healing practices are deeply ingrained within healthcare systems in many countries. In Bangladesh, these methods take center stage as primary forms of treatment, especially within the low socioeconomic communities and rural areas. Such healing practices have a spiritual foundation that incorporates healers such as Kalami and Bhandai that facilitate verses from holy books to invoke spirits to diagnose, provide treatment, and cure.[11] For individuals in middle or high socioeconomic status, they prefer modern healthcare practices but resort to traditional healers if modern treatments fail to cure the illness. In Bangladesh culture, a "good death" is one that takes place in the presences of spirits and loved ones.[12] It is important to highlight that most patients within the Bangladesh culture seek assistance from traditional healers and engage in spiritual practices. However, the timing and reasoning to turn to traditional healing may differ because of their own lived experiences and personal beliefs.

The perspective of dignity at the end of life in traditional Chinese culture was observed through interviews, and thematic analyses were conducted with fifteen advanced cancer patients and ten family members in China.[13] These patients suffered from physical and psychological distresses. The results showed that the meaning of dignity at the end of life in Chinese culture differed compared to Western culture. Chinese culture puts an emphasis on collectivism and importance of living in a moral way.[14] This means that one's dignity has a direct correlation to a cultur- ally specific dignity to live a stigma-free life; self-dignity, which means to live a healthy life with spiritual peace; family-related dignity, which means to not become a burden to the family; and care and treatment dignity, which means to be respected and make consent-based decisions.[15] However, in traditional Chinese culture, being diagnosed with a serious illness like cancer is perceived as a punishment for "being a bad person," which lowers the patient's dignity at end of life.[16] This leads to depression, anx- iety, and other forms of psychogenic pain within the patients due to the feeling of being a burden and losing the meaning and pur- pose of life. It is important to note that in Chinese culture, peace and dignity at end of life is evaluated through one's culture, indi- vidual perceptions of oneself, their family's perceptions, and the care and treatment received during their illness.

A VR therapist treating two such patients (one from Bangladesh and one from China) should not use the same methods but rather tailor the care to fit the patients' respective perception and narratives of life and death. Culture influences not only the type of healthcare preferences but is also associated with healing methods. For traditional Bangladesh patients, they may prefer traditional healing practices with a spiritual founda- tion at the end of life. To signify a good death in this culture, the presence of loved ones during transitions is a significant aspect. Therefore, the facilitator should consider incorporating spiritual elements within their treatment or facilitating in the presence of their loved ones. However, for traditional Chinese patients, they value respect, a consent-based decision-making process, and high-quality services. The Chinese culture perception of a good death is related to their dignity at end of life based on how morally correct they lived their lives before the illness. The facilitator should consider incorporating a high patient–physician rapport and ensuring the patient is guiding the care provided.

Meeting cultural and spiritual needs at the end of life and during serious illness is crucial as it nourishes the very essence of an individual's identity. Not meeting these needs causes an imbalance to the holistic approach of care that leads to a sense of discomfort and uncertainty, and hence increased psychogenic pain. When a VR therapist takes the time to understand the patient's culture and personal beliefs, it can lead to truly compassionate care. Aligning the treatment measures to the patient's values and beliefs can cause the patient to find clarity of their belonging to family or group and reduce the feeling of isolation. When patients are able to accept the illness and understand their purpose of life in the context of society, they are able to release the psychogenic pain and find inner peace.

For years, many healthcare systems have been designed to limit human interaction as the patient progresses through the stages of illness. Practitioners (or their insurers) tend to be more concerned with volume matters: how many patients are seen each day, each week, each month. Time matters, and how long a doctor is in a hospital room and not moving to the next is tracked, documentation is essential, and billing the right codes is critical—all of which take the practitioner's time away from each individual patient.

Specialty matters insofar as who serves in the primary care office versus who serves in the hospital inpatient setting. Many lucky people in the United States, because they have never been sick enough to be hospitalized, still do not realize, or understand that if admitted, they will likely not see the doctor whose office they chose or who they go to when sick with less critical ailments. Instead, their care will be guided by a hospitalist, whom they have likely never met. Hefty regulatory standards that demand more time documentation than facetime, competition in healthcare that mandates certain strategies outside of good patient care are required, drug company ownership over so much of what takes place in healthcare with all the lobbying dollars they put into political efforts, insurance companies that dictate more care allowance and denials than do the physicians who know their patients and others—these are all problems that indicate the system is falling apart. These demands negate the ability to focus on areas within spiritual and cultural healing. These issues have sterilized every area of healthcare more than the antiseptic used in patient rooms. The danger is in this level of disconnect. Our systemic failures have excluded the pieces that embrace what it means to be human from being a part of treatment.

There is a call for disruption, a call for bringing back the human condition and awareness of what it means to be a vulnerable patient and what it means to truly care for them. Patients need more than medication and procedures; they need a holistic approach to the care they are seeking. The holistic approach proposed in this literature includes that which goes beyond physiological healing. Virtual reality (VR) is a tool to evoke wonder and awe. Wonder is an emotion, critical for an immuno-compromised vulnerable patient. To have wonder is to have an openness for more and better understanding of the why behind life-limiting illnesses. It is what every patient deserves.

Virtual Reality in a Medical Setting

Daniel was a patient who had experienced the world of medicine his entire life; he considered himself a professional patient. He was born with the same disease as the elephant man; his body was deformed, but his spirit was bright. From birth, the healthcare system was a part of his daily life. Instead of regularly scheduled sports activities like there are for other kids, Daniel was facing yet another acute intervention to get him through the next phase of childhood and immobility.

Daniel was a seriously ill patient: 110 surgeries and thousands of hospitalizations throughout his short life; tumors on every organ requiring every specialty, therapy, and allied health; Medicaid case management and home care; research across the country on his very rare congenital illness. He lived and functioned seriously ill. Though his optimistic demeanor fought against the life-limiting elements in his illness, the reality was that it was just that: life limiting.

Daniel said his bed trapped him, held him hostage, robbed him of experience when he was at his sickest. His stamina did not allow him to keep up with friends. He could not go to the mountains and take long walks through nature. He could not ride a wave at a beautiful beach and be one with the ocean. He could not travel to unique areas and experience a landscape outside of his day-to-day routine. When he was his sickest, his pain held him hostage to necessary opioids to get him through the day. The opioids held him hostage to morning nausea and vomiting, to fatigue and fogginess all day. His infections held him hostage to necessary IV antibiotics. And later in his disease, with organs smothered by growing tumors, his system was held hostage to machines for breathing, dialysis, and nutritional support. He was held hostage to his disease for the vast majority of his 30 years.

Daniel found VR before it had grown into the space it is today. He saw the potential for two key goals:

◆ Escape: VR was an escape from that bed, an experience that no TV show, no other type of distraction could match. When he had the ad hoc device on his face, he was immersed in that experience. He was no longer present alongside those machines or in that room, chair, or bed. He was elsewhere.

◆ Wonder and Awe: This experience gave Daniel the openness he needed to see the purpose in his illness, to see himself as something very small in this world but very big in the purpose of this world. The ability to put your brain in that mindset when you are vulnerable and trapped is a gift.

Daniel experienced VR years before it was as advanced as it is today. But for many patients, the entrapment he experienced is as present now as it was years ago—and maybe even more so.

Even back then, he recognized that the future of modern medicine is to bring the patient into that mountain or ocean.

We have modernized medicine to treat disease more than ever before but very few of those modern techniques, from drugs causing adverse effects to infusions causing terrible reactions, from dialysis machines that cause lethargy and a whole other kind of illness to ventilators supporting longevity or a temporary fix—manage to provide a sense wonder and not awe. All those technologies have advanced inhibiting disease progression and supported longevity, but none have advanced being human, solving for quality of life, solving for the mental-health issues that come up when the control of your physiological self has been completely removed by life-limiting illness. VR fights for both. VR may disrupt the very disconnect between medicine and humanity.

Breaks, Barriers, Boundaries, and Innovation

We are living in a time when patients and people are desperate to find healing outside of what we have known. Troubled with more mental-health issues than ever before, both those who are well and those who are seriously ill are seeking mental healing from anxiety, depression, and other mental illnesses. There is movement in the alternative forms of healing—for example, in the arts. Authors of *Your Brain on Art* cite story after story where the arts have unique and specialized healing for ailments from chronic pain to prevention of generalized disease. These are the breakthroughs pushing the barriers created by our broken healthcare system and our growing aged and ill populations. We are charged with breaking down the walls that have created the aforementioned silos, sterility, and disappointment that is our current system.

As many have heard anecdotally, history may repeat itself. Back in the days of less modern medicine, important components of healing were relationships with the healers in the community and one's own supernatural beliefs. This has never been less true than it is today. Having someone known to facilitate healing becomes just as important as the tools the practitioner is using to heal. Why? Because the relationship prompts trust and perpetuates actions on the part of the patient to support healing. It may be a placebo affect but it is definitely a well-documented anomaly.

One unique study even shows that providers who can maintain a compassionate interface with a patient for a mere 40 seconds can take down the walls of lacking rapport and soothe significant anxiety in the patient for better outcomes. This same study focuses, however, on the inability for practitioners to engage with limited compassion because their learned response is to avoid empathy to attempt to prevent compassion fatigue. The very overwhelming nature of medicine and the role caregivers take demand the disconnect. The irony, however, is that this disconnect is not necessarily protective for the provider and may lead to increasing burnout anyway. A system is working against itself when being human is taken out of the room.[17]

Palliative Care

Three years ago, my kidneys went into distress from the diagnosis given at birth and now I am a dialysis patient. Dialysis treatment is three, sometime four days a week and it is a very tiring process I would not wish on anyone. I never imagined that this would be my life at 12 years of age. Like other kids, I had hopes, dreams, and plans. Now, however, my life is truly day-by-day as my organs are shutting down due to renal failure.

Hospice and palliative care has been the help we needed so I could be cared for at home and a breath of relief for my mom as she worries so much. When the symptoms of the disease become too much for my mom and me to manage at home, luckily, we can call the provider to arrange services.

This is the response from a young patient who was rescued by palliative care while continuing to receive his aggressive treatments.

Palliative care is a unique intervention that has been around much longer than some of the newer healing arts. Palliative care embodies the art of pain and symptom management coupled with the art of communication. If we are driven by a specialized medicine world where the nephrologist treats the kidney and the neurologist treats the brain, then likewise the palliative-care physician has an organ as well. That organ is artful discussion of disease and goals of care and an acute knowledge of how pain therapies can improve symptoms. This is what those providers study in their fellowships.

The definition of palliative care can be summarized as follows: Palliative care is an interdisciplinary team approach designed for individuals facing terminal or life-limiting illnesses, incurable conditions, or incapacitating injuries. It includes expert management of pain and symptoms, caregiver support, and care coordination. The primary objective is to improve the quality of life for both patients and their families by easing the suffering caused by the illness and its treatments. This holistic care addresses physical, psychosocial, and spiritual aspects of suffering, tailoring its focus to the individual's and family's needs. Palliative care is adaptable across healthcare settings, and the definition underscores the importance of healthcare providers receiving training in fundamental palliative skills, such as effective communication and discussions about goals of care.[18]

These specialists are acting like the ancient provider in developing rapport, with lengthier times spent with each patient. They are working on goals with the patients and families. They are disseminating all the information from other providers so that there is a captain paying attention to all organs and all needs. They are calling in the whole team and practicing an interdisciplinary review of the patient and to consider them as a whole human instead of just a disease, just an infection, just a less-than-perfect organ.

The whole person is defined, physiologically, spiritually, intellectually, and artfully.[19] These providers are a tool on the road to recovery from the dehumanization of healthcare; however, there is a vast shortage of palliative providers and an underuse of the specialty. Thus, more tools are needed to disrupt the sterile norm. These providers rely on interventions and interdisciplinary support. Here is the response from one young patient to such care.

A Spiritual Deficit

Spirituality by definition means to breathe.[20] To be spiritual is to be human. This has somehow been lost to the worlds of defined religions and higher powers. But there is meaning past that which is defined and understood as spiritual or religious. Thus, those looking at change in the focus of life or transition from life to death straight on have an inherent need to address and care for spirituality.

The population is evolving and technology is increasing. But one thing still remains the same: All humans are influenced by the need of the human condition for care, for touch, for other people.

When a patient seeks healthcare, they are seeking healing. Though it may only be for one organ of the body or one event, when a patient is diagnosed chronically or seriously ill, it is a natural progression to crave whole-body/whole-person healing from the professional and to include spirituality.

The white coat creates more of a professional divide for clinical workers. Clinicians put a proverbial mask on with their patients.[21] This creates a disconnect unless perhaps the professional decides to bring their own spiritual meaning to the patient and unmask the divide. Seeking spiritual solace during the patient experience is difficult. The patient feels vulnerable and potential embarrassment for the demise of physical/mental self. The ability for the healthcare industry to acknowledge and address vulnerability, meaning, and shame is as important as physical treatment. The ability to pursue compassion is a part of this. In circumstance where illness becomes death, it is even more important to find spirituality. Humanity and compassion must cross from professional to patient.[22]

Time is a luxury most professionals cannot afford. From regulations to documentation standards, most caregivers cannot afford the luxury of giving true care. Nurses need spirituality training to protect their patient's vulnerability, or a tool to make this easier. Though spirituality can be considered with utmost importance, there is an informality in spiritual assessment that does not address the heaviness of the needs not being met.

These unmet needs became more apparent in the early days of COVID where the personhoods of patients were not attended to, only the disease, infection, and resources. During the pandemic, a sick patient might have to have been dropped off at the emergency room alone. There was understaffing, sick staffing, a needed changed treatment model with severe isolation protocols and an uncontrollable number of unknowns. This major shift in the healthcare experience coupled with the mass exodus from the great resignation and the change in industries as we knew them put an even tighter strain on all the anxieties and stressors of a plagued system. This became a time that no one was prepared for and most were at least ill prepared for. We needed meaning more than ever before.

A large part of the moral distress experienced by frontline healthcare workers during the pandemic was due to the inability to do more for their COVID patients and the effects of watching their patients die without their loved ones by their side.[23] When a patient was taken to the hospital with COVID, they were forced to abandon their family and their advocate—potentially abandoning their voice. Breathless and coughing, unconscious and struggling as many COVID patients were, the patient could not tell their story, achieve their goals, or find any source of awe. Witnessing this firsthand, as caregivers did, meant burnout ensued. Thus, the demand for resuscitating humanity back into medicine became all the more vital.

There is an aim to broaden spiritual care because there are not always enough personnel to cover pastoral care/chaplains to address the many needs of the growing seriously ill.[24] This is not an abundant area of healthcare where all healthcare institutions employ a person of this sort. Thus, the discipline is lacking in availability to train and support professional caregivers and to support patients.

Best-practice healthcare standards integrate an interdisciplinary team approach into medicine. The spiritual component adds breadth and depth to the patient experience. It is an opportunity to support the clinical staff in treating the whole patient. A spiritual assessment deviates from the expected physiological questions to patient meaning, purpose, fears, alignment with values. When nurtured, all these components make us more able to exist with illness and decrease the worrisome threat of transition to another state.

Many of the best accreditation programs cite spiritual needs being met as vital.[25] They demand a proponent of spiritual service to define best practices. Even Medicare regulations for hospice benefit require a chaplain as part of the care team from necessary outreach, assessments, and documentation.

Providing spiritual care is recognized as key component of high-quality patient care. Thus, this should never be excluded from the care of the patient. Although healthcare workers might feel sufficient in this role, chaplains are specialists in this role and other healthcare workers are not specifically trained in this area. Many healthcare facilities have no spiritually trained staff, and certainly those who carry this staff do not provide it at the same level as, say, the nurse or other clinicians.[26]

Palliative care in best practice incorporates spiritual care being a large focus. When the spiritual well-being of a patient is ignored, their overall quality of life is seen to diminish. Specialists excel in one area of the body, one organ—but our human body is a multifaceted, complex system. Physicians are understandably trained to focus on one facet, giving them more skill and knowledge of that area. Unfortunately, this focus can cause them to lose the ability to see the whole picture of a patient, and they particularly miss the existential and spiritual pain that comes along with disease or illness. As we show in the case studies in this book, it is important that this area of care is provided by a specialist who is trained in spiritual care and has the experience to understand a patient's spiritual needs and the ability to provide the support needed. This type of knowledge comes from experience and training. When spiritual needs are addressed by healthcare generalists who are not equipped to handle these situations, the outcome is not as positive. One study found that out of the 489 patients surveyed, the ones visited by a chaplain compared to generalists had far better outcomes, reporting overall satisfaction, and feeling that their nonphysical needs (emotional and spiritual) had been met.[27]

Professionals, especially experts in palliative care, shared in one study the absolute importance those with the most experience in the profession maintained *all* patients must pursue spiritual healing for closure. Such treatment is necessary for security in illness.[28] Illness, especially terminal illness, brings about many feelings for a patient; anxiety, insecurity, depression and feelings of loss of their future. As with any illness, thoughts of the future and what that might look like with disease and treatment can be extremely overwhelming. Diagnosis of any kind could have an impact on a person's quality of life. These situations are delicate and best handled by healthcare professionals trained in providing spiritual guidance and comfort.

The Caregiver Population Too

To be a caregiver is to suffer. A "sandwiched" caregiver is one who is living with parents who act childish and need childish attention but who also has children who require the same. The pull is great to address the suffering, to fix the pain, to do well by them all. As an aging and debilitated population emerges, this will occur even more often. If we do not address the suffering of both those whose disease and frailty have increased and those who care for them with tools to help, our majority population may whither from the strain, from the mental-health anguish, from the lapse in bodily control. They need well-guided tools to ease the struggle.[29] Caregivers can likewise benefit from the VR therapy experience. There is growing need for the caregiver population from the family, as the number of professional caregivers is limited. Thus, it becomes more important to take care of those caregivers so they may continue on as the aging population continues to expand.

Approximately one in five Americans, or 53 million people, have provided care to a disabled or sick loved one in the past year.[30] Data shows that women make up around 61% of caregivers and nearly 90% of the care is given to a relative.[31] As a caregiver, the time commitment, financial, physical, and emotional burden is equivalent to having a part-time job.[32] In a different study, using the Blue Cross Blue Shield data, it was estimated that 51 million Americans require a caregiver.[33]

Technology in Healthcare

New technologies are emerging almost daily, and almost all of them require more trained personnel. For example, the dialysis machine and the ventilator have both improved longevity and the ability to weather an acute patient event or illness storm. However, their introduction has required new caregivers in medicine. Respiratory therapists are the discipline who manage breathing technologies. Dialysis units and nurses are those who manage these machines. These two examples align heightened technology with the need for people. VR is not unique in this way. To place a device on a patient without prompting, directions, instruction, and a meaningful conversation is not to achieve the goal of success found in the case studies of Chapter 1. The facilitator is a very important proponent to a successful VR experience.

On the flip side of that coin is the introduction of AI into healthcare. With additional intuitive and intelligence, this may introduce a first technology where fewer people are needed to be caregivers. This presents an opportunity for professional caregivers to go back to the roots of what it means to care and be at the bedside and to address what it is to see someone feeling bad and make them feel better.

Mark Aulisio argues that technology in AI will potentially steal away the roles of the caregiver and give them back their ability and desire to care for the human, at the bedside without all the horrendous bells and whistles of the EMR and the rest of the drag that added healthcare has brought.[34] As an example, if the nurse no longer has to focus on laborious and tedious documentation because the AI puts this documentation together for them, then areas of true patient care—to listen, to advise, to teach, and to empathize—will be available. VR can help mend that gap by providing a tool for the professional caregiver to utilize.

VR opens up those conversations between professional caregiver and patient, removing the patient from the sterile environment and placing them into a world of awe and meaning so as to have the opportunity to reflect on the purpose of life and the experience of having a life-limiting illness. These programs breathe relaxation into the patient. Perhaps it will be VR in serious illness that breathes life back into the humanity of healthcare. This technology will alleviate the suffering of the ill held hostage by their situation and the professional caregivers held hostage by defense mechanisms and burnout. It will provide a spiritual tool for those who have not been approached or helped by any spiritual closure or nurturing during their journey. Most vitally, it will provide a gateway to find wonder and awe to those who have lost this in their life, potentially with some permanence.

References

1 Gunja, M.Z., Gumas, E.D., & Williams II, R.D. (2023). *U.S. health care from a global perspective, 2022: Accelerating spending, worsening outcomes* (Commonwealth Fund). https://doi.org/10.26099/8ejy-yc74

2 Johnson, M., Albizri, A., & Harfouche, A. (2021). Responsible artificial intelligence in healthcare: Predicting and preventing insurance claim denials for economic and social wellbeing. *Information Systems Frontiers, 25*(6), 2179–2195. https://doi.org/10.1007/s10796-021-10137-5

3 Mirmirani, S., & Spivack, R.N. (1993). Health care system collapse in the United States: Capitalist market failure! *De Economist, 141*(3), 419–431.

4 Mirmirani, S., & Spivack, R.N. (1993). Health care system collapse in the United States: Capitalist market failure! *De Economist, 141*(3), 419–431.

5 Mirmirani, S., & Spivack, R.N. (1993). Health care system collapse in the United States: Capitalist market failure! *De Economist, 141*(3), 419–431.

6 Vespa, J. (2018). The U.S. joins other countries with large aging populations. *United States Census Bureau*. Retrieved from https://www.census.gov/library/stories/2018/03/graying-america.html

7 World Health Organization. (2022, October 1). Ageing and health. Retrieved from https://www.who.int/news-room/fact-sheets/detail/ageing-and-health

8 Speck, P. (2016). Culture and spirituality: Essential components of palliative care. *Postgraduate Medical Journal, 92*(1088), 341–345. https://doi.org/10.1136/postgradmedj-2015-33369

9 Speck, P. (2016). Culture and spirituality: Essential components of palliative care. *Postgraduate Medical Journal, 92*(1088), 341–345. https://doi.org/10.1136/postgradmedj-2015-33369

10 Speck, P. (2016). Culture and spirituality: Essential components of palliative care. *Postgraduate Medical Journal, 92*(1088), 341–345. https://doi.org/10.1136/postgradmedj-2015-33369

11 Haque, Md.I., Chowdhury, A.B., Shahjahan, M., & Harun, Md.G. (2018). Traditional healing practices in rural Bangladesh: A qualitative investigation. *BMC Complementary and Alternative Medicine, 18*(1). https://doi.org/10.1186/s12906-018-2129-5

12 Haque, Md.I., Chowdhury, A.B., Shahjahan, Md., & Harun, Md.G. (2018). Traditional healing practices in rural Bangladesh: A qualitative investigation. *BMC Complementary and Alternative Medicine, 18*(1). https://doi.org/10.1186/s12906-018-2129-5

13 Liu, L., Ma, L., Chen, Z., Geng, H., Xi, L., McClement, S., & Guo, Q. (2021). Dignity at the end of life in traditional Chinese culture: Perspectives of Advanced cancer patients and family members. *European Journal of Oncology Nursing, 54*, 102017. https://doi.org/10.1016/j.ejon.2021.102017

14 Liu, L., Ma, L., Chen, Z., Geng, H., Xi, L., McClement, S., & Guo, Q. (2021). Dignity at the end of life in traditional Chinese culture: Perspectives of advanced cancer patients and family members. *European Journal of Oncology Nursing, 54*, 102017. https://doi.org/10.1016/j.ejon.2021.102017

15 Liu, L., Ma, L., Chen, Z., Geng, H., Xi, L., McClement, S., & Guo, Q. (2021). Dignity at the end of life in traditional Chinese culture: Perspectives of advanced cancer patients and family members. *European Journal of Oncology Nursing, 54*, 102017. https://doi.org/10.1016/j.ejon.2021.102017

16 Liu, L., Ma, L., Chen, Z., Geng, H., Xi, L., McClement, S., & Guo, Q. (2021). Dignity at the end of life in traditional Chinese culture: Perspectives of advanced cancer patients and family members. *European*

Journal of Oncology Nursing, 54, 102017. https://doi.org/10.1016/j.ejon.2021.102017

17 Llorente-Barroso, C., Kolotouchkina, O., & Mañas-Viniegra, L. (2021). The enabling role of ICT to mitigate the negative effects of emotional and social loneliness of the elderly during COVID-19 pandemic. *International Journal of Environmental Research in Public Health, 18*, 3923. https://doi.org/10.3390/ ijerph18083923

18 Michigan HomeCare & Hospice Association. (2023, January). *The State of Palliative Care in Michigan*. [Meeting Minutes].

19 Magsamen, S., & Ross, I. (2023). *Your brain on art: How the arts transform us*. New York: Random House.

20 García-Navarro, E.B., Medina-Ortega, A., & García Navarro, S. (2021). Spirituality in patients at the end of life—is it necessary? A qualitative approach to the protagonists. *International Journal of Environmental Research and Public Health, 19*(1), 227.

21 Condon, P. & Makransky, J. (2021). Compassion practices. In D. Rakel & V. Minichiello (eds.), *Integrative Medicine* (5th ed.). New York: Elsevier.

22 DeFord, B. (2023). The personal and the professional: Mindfulness, spiritual life and health care [article under review]. The spiritual cycle of providing professional health care. *OBM Integrated and Complementary Medicine, 8*(1).

23 Norman, S.B., Feingold, J.H., Kaye-Kauderer, H., Kaplan, C.A., Hurtado, A., Kachadourian, L., et al. (2021). Moral distress in frontline healthcare workers in the initial epicenter of the COVID-19 pandemic in the United States: Relationship to PTSD symptoms, burnout, and psychosocial functioning. *Depression and Anxiety, 38*(10), 1007–1017.

24 Batstone, E., Bailey, C., & Hallett, N. (2020). Spiritual care provision to end-of-life patients: A systematic literature review. *Journal of Clinical Nursing, 29*(19–20), 3609–3624.

25 McCurry, I., Jennett, P., Oh, J., White, B., & DeLisser, H.M. (2021). Chaplain care in the intensive care unit at the end of life: A qualitative analysis. *Palliative Medicine Reports, 2*(1), 280–286.

26 Taylor, E.J., Mamier, I., Ricci-Allegra, P., & Foith, J. (2017). Self-reported frequency of nurse-provided spiritual care. *Applied Nursing Research, 35*, 30–35.

27 Benton, K., Zerbo, K.R., Decker, M., & Buck, B. (2019). Development and Evaluation of an outpatient palliative care clinic. *Journal*

of *Hospice and Palliative Nursing*, *21*(2), 160–166. https://doi.org/10.1097/NJH.0000000000000544

28 Pentaris, P., & Tripathi, K. (2022). Palliative professionals' views on the importance of religion, belief, and spiritual identities toward the end of life. *International Journal of Environmental Research and Public Health*, *19*(10), 6031.

29 World Health Organization. (2022, October 1). Ageing and health. Retrieved from https://www.who.int/news-room/fact-sheets/detail/ageing-and-health; House Study Committee on Expanding Long-Term Care Options; HR 141 (2023). Retrieved from https://www.legis.ga.gov/api/legislation/document/20232024/214064

30 Jean-Louis, F. (2022, July 28). *Family caregiver burden grows as the population ages*. Addressing the growing family caregiver burden, RTI Health Advance. Retrieved from https://healthcare.rti.org/insights/family-caregiver-burden-growing-with-aging-population

31 Jean-Louis, F. (2022, July 28). *Family caregiver burden grows as the population ages*. Addressing the growing family caregiver burden, RTI Health Advance. Retrieved from https://healthcare.rti.org/insights/family-caregiver-burden-growing-with-aging-population

32 Jean-Louis, F. (2022, July 28). *Family caregiver burden grows as the population ages*. Addressing the growing family caregiver burden, RTI Health Advance. Retrieved from https://healthcare.rti.org/insights/family-caregiver-burden-growing-with-aging-population

33 The Economic Impact of Caregiving. (2021). Blue cross blue shield. Retrieved from https://www.bcbs.com/the-health-of-america/reports/the-economic-impact-of-caregiving

34 Mark Aulisio (personal communication, August 8, 2023).

3

The Application of VR in Mental-Health Care

Yee Hui Yeo and Brennan Spiegel

The Burden of Mental-Health Disorders

The global landscape of mental and addictive disorders is characterized by its extensive reach, impacting over 1 billion individuals worldwide.[1] This prevalence not only signifies a substantial health concern but also poses a significant economic challenge,[2] with further exacerbation during the COVID-19 pandemic.[3]

Within the United States, the prevalence of mental-health disorders presents a concerning picture. In 2023, approximately 21% of the adult population, translating to 50 million Americans, reported experiencing a mental-health illness.[4] Specifically, it is projected that 9.5% of adult Americans will experience a depressive disorder, while around 18% are expected to suffer from an anxiety disorder.[5] Additionally, 15.35% of adults and 6.34% of youth reported having a substance use disorder (SUD) in 2023.[6]

DOI: 10.4324/9781032649771-3

Treatment of Anxiety Disorder, Depression, and Substance Use Disorder

The ultimate goal of initial treatment in anxiety disorder and depression is to reach a state of remission, which is essentially the resolution of the anxiety or depressive syndrome, while the goal was cessation for SUDs.[7] Pharmacotherapy, alongside cognitive-behavioral therapy (CBT), emerges as effective initial option for the treatment of anxiety disorders and major depression.[8] CBT, a widely recognized form of psychotherapy, plays a crucial role in managing mental-health disorders.[9] It involves challenging and restructuring the patient's overarching and individual belief systems, as well as associated behaviors, to alleviate presenting symptoms. CBT is particularly prominent in the treatment of anxiety disorders, supported by substantial evidence from meta-analyses demonstrating its effectiveness.[10] In the context of depression, CBT has demonstrated greater efficacy compared to control conditions like waiting lists or no treatment at all.[11] Turning to SUDs, particularly alcohol use, motivational interviewing has emerged as a mainstream intervention.[12] Defined as a client-oriented counseling style, it assists clients in exploring and resolving ambivalence toward change. This approach is particularly impactful in reducing alcohol use, as evidenced by its effectiveness across various populations, whether delivered individually by therapists or in a group setting, though the latter requires further evaluation.[13] A meta-analysis encompassing 12 studies with 1,721 patients revealed that a combination of CBT and motivational interviewing for patients with clinical or subclinical depressive and alcohol use disorders yields a slight but clinically significant improvement in treatment outcomes.[14] Combined pharmacotherapy and psychotherapy are recommended over the exclusive use of either pharmacotherapy or psychotherapy.[15]

The Role of Telemedicine in Psychotherapy

Telemedicine, defined as the use of telecommunications and information technologies to provide health information and services across geographical distances,[16] has significantly enhanced access to psychotherapy.[17] Telemedicine offers increased convenience for clients regarding appointment locations and flexible timing, making it a more accessible option for many.[18] Its adoption, increasing since the early 1990s, has been substantiated by seminal studies, including a 1995 study demonstrating its effectiveness in treating panic disorder with agoraphobia compared to a wait-list comparison group,[19] and later trials for patients with obsessive-compulsive disorder[20] and for elderly patients with anxiety disorders.[21]

However, challenges in building a therapeutic alliance due to the absence of nonauditory cues and a potential lack of attentiveness from patients are notable.[22] Furthermore, randomized controlled trials (RCTs) suggest that options like videoconferencing can reduce treatment dropouts and extend treatment courses.[23] On a broader scheme, the SUPPORT for Patients and Communities Act contains provisions that endorse the further use of telemedicine for SUD.[24] The use of telemedicine in mental-health care was profoundly boosted during the COVID-19 pandemic. Platforms like BetterHelp, which connect clients with licensed professionals in distant regions, have expanded the reach of mental-health services, allowing individuals access to a wider variety of practitioners through messaging, phone, or videoconference.[25] Additionally, Alcoholics Anonymous meetings and other support services like the Substance Abuse and Mental Health Service Administration (SAMHSA, https://www.samhsa.gov/) have adapted to online formats to decrease barriers to accessing conventional in-person meetings (https://www.aa.org/).

Undertreatment of Mental-Health Disorder

Despite these advancements in telemedicine, which have improved the feasibility and accessibility of treatment, the scarcity of trained clinicians remains a pressing issue, emphasizing the need for continued focus on training and development in telemedicine-based psychotherapy. The undertreatment of mental-health disorders remains a significant concern, as highlighted by the fact that over half (54.7%) of adults with mental illness receive no treatment, and this figure is even more alarming in those with substance use disorder (SUD), where 93.5% did not receive treatment.[26] Despite the increasing availability and convenience of pharmacotherapy,[27] significant barriers persist in accessing and continuing treatment. Structural barriers such as the cost of treatment, limited insurance coverage, difficulties in finding appropriate care, and challenges in attending appointments,[28] coupled with attitudinal barriers like perceptions about the necessity and effectiveness of treatment, a belief in handling problems independently, and stigma, contribute to the low rate of treatment.[29]

The Role of Virtual Reality in Mental-Health Disorders

Virtual reality (VR), a computer-generated simulation of three-dimensional environments, offers a groundbreaking method for delivering mental-health support. VR immerses users in an interactive virtual space, typically through head-mounted displays (HMDs) or multi-projected environments, creating realistic images, sounds, and other sensations. This immersive experience can stimulate visual, auditory, tactile, and even olfactory senses, leading to a heightened sense of presence and memory engagement in these virtual settings.[30] The technology's ability to create place and plausibility illusions results in realistic behavior within immersive virtual environments.[31] This aspect of VR has significant therapeutic potential, particularly in psychiatric disorders. It is being employed to treat conditions such as anxiety disorders, posttraumatic stress disorder (PTSD), phobias, psychosis, depression, eating disorders, and SUDs. Research suggests that VR can safely and effectively recreate challenging scenarios, allowing individuals to practice and refine appropriate responses based on theoretical understandings of specific disorders.[32] These simulations, which can be adjusted in difficulty and repeated as needed, enable individuals to confront difficult situations in a virtual context before transferring these learnings to real-world settings. Next, we focus on the main theme of this chapter: anxiety disorder, depression, and SUDs.

The Application of VR in Anxiety Disorder and Depression

The immersive and interactive nature of VR provides a unique and effective approach for patients with anxiety disorder and depression. During VR exposure therapy, patients are equipped with relaxation and coping strategies, such as breathing relaxation or cognitive restructuring, to assist them through the treatment process. This is particularly pertinent in the treatment of phobias and anxiety, where patients progress at an individual pace through a graded exposure hierarchy, repeating steps until a significant decrease in anxiety is achieved. The cognitive and behavioral theories underpinning VR's use in therapeutic settings suggested by a previous study, Behavioral Framework of Immersive Technologies (BehaveFIT), are pivotal.[33] They demonstrate how VR's immersive characteristics can influence cognitive processes and behavior change, drawing on the social cognitive theory and the theory of planned behavior. This framework underscores VR's ability to create realistic, engaging environments that can be used to modify cognitive schemas and behavior patterns. Moreover, the controllable and customizable nature of VR environments makes them adaptable to various age groups, cultural backgrounds, and severity of psychological conditions. Finally, VR has shown promise in enhancing patient engagement and adherence to standard treatments. Incorporating elements like gamification and persuasive technology into VR interventions holds great potential to keep users engaged and motivated, particularly in the treatment of anxiety and depression.[34] This adaptability and engagement factor of VR in mental-health care not only broadens its applicability but also enhances its effectiveness, representing a significant advancement in the field.

Historically, the use of VR in mental health began with experimental stages focusing on anxiety management techniques (AMT) for treating phobias. Early applications included treatments for spider phobia,[35] fear of heights,[36] fear of flying,[37] and claustrophobia.[38] VR's effectiveness extended to other conditions like posttraumatic stress disorder.[39] Moreover, some studies have demonstrated a long-lasting positive impact on patients' real-life experiences.[40] Although the initial evidence, primarily from case reports, was of low quality, the landscape of VR in mental health has evolved significantly. Since the early 2010s, more robust research, including RCTs, has emerged, particularly in areas like social anxiety.[41] This evolution marks a transition from VR being a novel experimental approach to a validated therapeutic tool with a growing body of high-quality evidence supporting its efficacy in various mental-health conditions.

Studies on Anxiety Disorder

In the field of anxiety disorders, the application of VR in exposure therapy represents a significant advancement. Exposure therapy, long considered the most effective treatment for anxiety disorders, often encounters challenges such as exacerbating patients' anxiety or limitations in exposing patients to the actual source of fear. VR therapy offers a safer alternative, enabling patients to experience anxiety-inducing environments virtually. The integration of wearable devices during VR sessions allows for the objective measurement of bio-signal data, such as heart rate and galvanic skin reflex, providing valuable insights into the patient's physiological response to anxiety.[42]

Real-time monitoring of bio-signals related to anxiety during VR therapy facilitates a more controlled and logical increase in exposure to anxiety-inducing stimuli. For instance, studies have demonstrated VR exposure therapy's effectiveness in reducing symptoms of acrophobia (fear of heights). A meta-analysis on aerophobia revealed that VR exposure therapy (VRE) not only paralleled the results of traditional therapies but also yielded better outcomes posttreatment and during follow-up periods.[43] The tailored environments of VRE have led to its active use in specific phobias, garnering higher patient preferences (76%) and lower treatment rejections compared to in vivo exposure treatment.[44]

While there is some heterogeneity and potential for publication bias in existing research, previous meta-analysis has shown that VR interventions generally outperform control conditions in treating anxiety.[45] A meta-analysis showed that VRE-based CBT (VRE-CBT) was as effective as CBT for severe anxiety disorders.[46] An early meta-analysis highlighted VR's substantial effect compared to control conditions in the field of anxiety, noting a dose-dependent response and the ability to transfer these effects to real-life situations.[47]

Further research, such as a systematic review and meta-analysis on VR-assisted CBT for anxiety disorders[48] and a meta-analysis on the effectiveness of VR exposure-based CBT for severe anxiety disorders, OCD, and PTSD,[49] reinforce these findings. Moreover, it's not just the stimuli provided by VR that are impactful but also the content within the VR environment. For example, a study showed that gaming on an immersive VR platform led to the amelioration of anxiety in patients with congenital heart disease, underscoring the multifaceted potential of VR in treating various aspects of anxiety disorders (PMID: 38234943).[50]

Studies on Posttraumatic Stress Disorder

VR-based therapies have emerged as a promising approach for treating posttraumatic stress disorder (PTSD), addressing various traumatic experiences such as war, terrorist attacks, violent assaults, and motor vehicle accidents. The recreation of these traumatic situations in the real world is challenging, making VR an ideal alternative. In VR-based therapies, patients predominantly passively narrate their trauma while visually exploring the virtual environment (VE) through an HMD. Therapists play a crucial role by adapting the VE in real time through a control panel, based on the patient's description of the traumatic event.[51] This adaptation involves manipulating anxiety-provoking stimuli, which may include visual, auditory, olfactory, or tactile elements, to effectively trigger stressful reactions and access the fear memory.

Patients with PTSD often report feeling safer in a VR environment compared to real-life situations, with a preference for VR therapy.[52] For instance, in treating victims of motor vehicle accidents, VR setups resemble real-life roads and include elements like a steering wheel and pedals, with visual, auditory, and tactile stimuli used to alter anxiety levels. During these sessions, therapists can modify parameters such as traffic density, time of day, weather conditions, and specific driving events, leading to significant improvements in posttrauma symptoms including reexperiencing, avoidance, and emotional numbing.[53]

Incorporating gamification and personalization has also proven effective. One study used a personalized truck-driving simulator as an action-cue exposure therapy for truck drivers with PTSD.[54] Similarly, a gaming-style design involving a virtual Huey helicopter flying over a virtual Vietnam was used for Vietnam combat veterans with PTSD, complete with realistic sounds of gunshots and explosions.[55] Additionally, a study implementing VR-graded exposure therapy (VR-GET) for combat-related PTSD integrated meditation for facilitating emotional, cognitive, and physical relaxation, resulting in marked reductions in PTSD symptom severity defined using PHQ-9, PTSD Checklist for DSM-5, and Beck Anxiety Inventory.[56] Another poignant example includes recreating the 9/11 World Trade Center attack, with jets crashing into the towers and animated explosions, for survivors who developed acute PTSD.[57]

However, it is noteworthy that an RCT found prolonged exposure to be more efficacious than VR exposure treatment for active-duty Army soldiers with PTSD from deployments to Iraq or Afghanistan.[58] Despite this, the dropout rates were high for both VR exposure therapy (VRE) and prolonged exposure (PE). A meta-analysis on VR-based graded exposure therapy in PTSD patients reported significant decreases in PTSD and depression symptoms posttreatment.[59]

These findings suggest that while VR-based therapies for PTSD offer innovative and effective treatment options, they may not universally outperform traditional exposure therapies. The evolving landscape of VR in PTSD treatment highlights its potential as a supplementary or alternative method, especially in cases where traditional exposure therapy is not feasible or less preferred by patients.

Depression

In the realm of depression treatment, the evidence supporting the use of VR is still emerging, but several innovative studies have begun to explore its potential. Falconer and colleagues focused on employing VR to treat depressive symptoms by fostering self-compassion and diminishing self-criticism.[60] This study demonstrated a reduction in depressive symptoms within four weeks, with around 40% of participants experiencing a clinically significant reduction.

In contrast, a novel study assessing VR cognitive training in a real-life virtual supermarket setting for depressed patients did not find substantial benefits (https://www.sciencedirect .com/science/article/abs/pii/S0747563217305927).[61] Patients practiced learning and purchasing shopping-list products in a VE, but the VR therapy did not show a distinct advantage in training performance, recognition, performance speed, spatial orientation, self-perceived daily cognitive impairments, real-life shopping tasks, or various neuropsychological capabilities compared to traditional desktop-based training.

Another intriguing approach involved the creation of virtual images and environments, such as a garden, tailored for senior users.[62] The objective was to evoke the belief and feeling of being in a real environment, aiming to improve the quality of life for elderly individuals with depression.

A study focused on postnatal depression explored the feasibility of combining CBT with VR.[63] While the combination showed potential, it also highlighted limitations and technical challenges that need addressing. Additionally, a VR-based stress management program for individuals with mood disorders, involving daily sessions of psychoeducation and VR-based relaxation practice, demonstrated significant reductions in scores on the Depression, Anxiety, and Stress Scale (DASS-21).[64] Moreover, an innovative study found that VR dance exercise was associated with a significant reduction in the Beck Depression Inventory score after six weeks of treatment, indicating the diverse applications and benefits of VR in depression therapy.[65]

These studies collectively suggest that while VR's role in treating depression is still in its formative stages, it holds promise, especially in creating tailored, immersive environments that can support traditional therapeutic methods.

The Application of VR in Substance Use Disorders

In the treatment of SUDs, VR is being increasingly explored due to its unique ability to address the chronic and repetitive over-stimulation of dopamine pathways, which is a fundamental trigger of addiction. Craving, a key factor in the development and maintenance of SUDs, is often initiated and exacerbated by social and environmental contexts that recall drug and alcohol consumption.[66] Studies have shown that interventions targeting sensitivity and reactivity to these environmental contexts and cues are essential to complement pharmacotherapy in treating SUDs (PMID: 20837060).[67]

Customized VR environments can effectively elicit strong cravings, making them useful in reducing these cravings when integrated with standard treatments.[68] Unlike traditional cue exposure methods that might use photographs or videos, VR can recreate social and environmental contexts in a more immersive and realistic way, thereby inducing cravings that closely resemble those experienced in real life.[69] The basis of cue exposure therapy in VR lies in the principle of classical conditioning, where a neutral cue, after being paired with an unconditioned stimulus, evokes a conditioned response similar to the unconditioned response.[70] This concept is key to understanding persistent substance use and abuse. VR environments have been shown to evoke cravings more effectively than two-dimensional cues. For instance, early studies using a nicotine craving questionnaire and fMRI scans revealed that VR environments triggered significant brain activity changes in regions associated with craving.[71]

Specific studies have demonstrated VR's effectiveness in various aspects of SUD treatment. One study showed that VR could induce different patterns of subjective craving for cigarettes, with smoking-related environments causing a more rapid increase in craving intensity.[72] Another found that VR environments, especially when combined with olfactory stimuli, significantly increased cravings in smokers regardless of their abstinence state.[73] VR has also been used to induce alcohol cravings, with binge drinkers experiencing higher cravings than non-binge drinkers.[74]

In the treatment of alcohol use disorder (AUD), patients undergoing VR therapy exhibited a greater decrease in craving after ten treatment sessions compared to those receiving CBT.[75] This indicates that VR could serve as both a treatment adjunct and an evaluation tool for identifying high-risk patients. Additionally, VR allows patients to confront triggers in simulated environments and practice coping strategies, tuning down craving intensity and addressing substance use in SUDs.

An RCT demonstrated VR's effectiveness in reducing cravings and improving physiological responses in alcohol-dependent patients during cue exposure.[76] From another angle, a clinical trial examined VR's effectiveness in training inexperienced volunteers in drug use prevention, enhancing their problem-solving abilities, self-efficacy, and teamwork.[77]

These findings collectively suggest that VR holds significant potential as a therapeutic tool in SUD treatment, offering innovative ways to confront and manage cravings and providing valuable training for both patients and those involved in addiction support and prevention.

Factors That Could Affect the Efficacy of VR-Based Therapy

In addition to the content of the therapy, several factors can significantly influence its efficacy.

1. **Novelty factor**: One such factor is the novelty of the technology. When users engage with VR for the first time, the novelty factor, as outlined by Peixoto and colleagues, can heighten their interest in using the headset.[78] However, this same novelty might also

detract from their attention and focus on the therapeutic aspects of the experience, potentially diminishing the therapy's effectiveness.

2. **Immersive tendencies**: This refers to an individual's inherent ability to become deeply engaged in a VE, playing a crucial role in the effectiveness of VR therapy. This concept encompasses cognitive, emotional, and imaginative aspects, allowing for an increased focus and reduced susceptibility to external distractions. Individuals with higher immersive tendencies are likely to engage more profoundly with the VR environment, potentially leading to more realistic emotional responses and enhancing the therapy's realism and effectiveness.

3. **The degree of realism**: Realism in VR is about accurately representing situations in a way that is true to life, providing an immersive experience that captures the user's entire field of vision, as opposed to traditional two-dimensional screens. Enhanced realism can contribute to a greater sense of place and plausibility illusion, increasing patient engagement with the simulated environment during therapy sessions. This improved realism may directly correlate with the therapeutic outcomes, as patients might feel more connected to and impacted by the VR experience.

4. **Enhanced interaction**: Finally, enhanced interaction within VR environments, particularly through artificial intelligence (AI)–driven conversational agents (CAs) and virtual companions, can significantly impact the therapy's success. These interactive elements provide assistance and companionship, creating a more engaging and supportive environment for users. From facilitating conversations to offering guidance, these AI elements can enrich the VR experience, making it more interactive and socially dynamic.

In our next section, we comprehensively review the development of AI-operated CAs and its integration into VR to enhance the treatment of anxiety disorder, depression, and SUD.

Application of AI-operated Conversational Agent in Providing Mental-Health Support

The integration of AI-operated CAs in mental-health care represents a significant evolution in the field.[79] These advancements in natural language processing and machine learning have opened new avenues for diagnosing, treating, and supporting mental resilience.[80] For example, large language models (LLMs) such as ChatGPT (OpenAI) or its newer version, GPT-4, as well as Gemini (Google), and Claude (Anthropic), are proliferating. ChatGPT, an advanced LLM, trained on diverse datasets and fine-tuned with RLHF, shows proficiency in clinical scenarios.[81] GPT-4, its successor, further enhances this performance.[82] The increasing use of CAs in healthcare, especially those operated by LLMs, as evidenced by growing research and commercial interest, indicates a shift toward more technologically advanced treatment methods.

Smartphone and tablet applications have emerged as the most popular platforms for delivering CA interventions. A systematic review and meta-analysis highlighted that CAs are effective in improving conditions like depression, distress, stress, and acrophobia.[83] However, their impact on subjective psychological well-being was not statistically significant, though they were generally found to be safe in mental-health contexts. Another meta-analysis demonstrated that conversational agents could effectively alleviate psychological distress, particularly when employing generative AI, using multimodal or voice-based CAs, or delivering interventions via mobile applications and instant messaging platforms.[84] The key factors influencing user experiences included the therapeutic relationship with the CA, content quality, and preventing communication breakdowns.

Further, a randomized control trial comparing the effectiveness of an app versus an AI CA-based intervention for SUD revealed the CA's superiority in aspects like positivity, personalization, and insight into drinking behaviors.[85] A notable study assessing the efficacy of an AI CA named "Tess" among college students found significant reductions in self-identified symptoms of depression and anxiety.[86] The RCT involved participants from various universities and used validated scales like the PHQ-9, GAD-7, and PANAS for evaluation. Participants interacting with Tess showed significant symptom improvement compared to the control group, illustrating the potential of AI CAs as cost-effective, supplementary mental-health support.

Woebot, another conversational agent, has shown effectiveness in immediate, empathetic patient response using CBT principles.[87] Studies involving Woebot for SUDs and mood & anxiety disorders reported significant reductions in substance use and improvements in mental-health metrics like the PHQ-8 and GAD-7.[88] Another digital mental-health intervention, Wysa, a multi-component mobile app using CA technology and text-based access to human counselors, has been beneficial in orthopedic patients with elevated depression or anxiety symptoms. Users showed improvements in PROMIS Depression, Pain Interference, and Physical Function scores.[89]

These findings underscore the growing importance and potential of AI-driven CAs in mental-health care, offering innovative, accessible, and effective solutions for managing various mental-health conditions, including anxiety, depression, and SUDs. Having explored the multifaceted applications and benefits of both VR and AI-operated CAs in mental health, we now turn our focus to the next frontier in this technological evolution: the integration of AI-operated CAs into VR environments.

Incorporating AI-operated CA into Virtual Reality

The integration of AI-operated CAs with VR marks a significant development in mental-health treatment, heralding a new era of immersive, interactive, and personalized therapy experiences. Theoretically, embedding AI-driven CAs in VR allows dynamic interactions that mimic real-life scenarios and provide tailored therapy. This amalgamation enhances therapy's realism and leverages AI-operated CAs' nuanced understanding and empathetic responses.

Before ChatGPT's widespread use, AI and VR integration was proposed in industrial applications by Trappey et al. for transformer design and manufacturing.[90] The AI component, based on a retrieval-based Q&A system, was trained on a large dataset for natural language understanding. The VR aspect allows for immersive visualization of transformers, aiding in design consultation and decision-making. This integration exemplifies the potential of AI and VR in industrial applications, offering efficient, interactive, and customer-centric solutions.

Since the release of LLMs such as ChatGPT, there have been ongoing efforts to integrate LLM into VR. An article on AI technologies like ChatGPT and DALL-E in the metaverse exemplifies this, showing AI's role in creating detailed environments and characters, thus revolutionizing digital experiences.[91] In this section, we explore how this integration transforms mental-health interventions, offering customization and adaptability for individual needs, particularly in anxiety disorders, depression, and SUDs. The potential of AI-enabled CAs within VR to provide continuous support and adaptive learning opens new doors for innovative treatment strategies. There is little evidence in the literature about the implementation and efficacy of this new technology. Herein, we present two in-house studies incorporating a GPT-4-enabled AI therapist in VR for anxiety, depression, and SUDs, demonstrating ChatGPT's capabilities.

Anxiety and Depression

As mentioned above, the fusion of VR and LLMs, such as GPT-4, heralds a new era of therapeutic possibilities in the realm of mental-health care. This synergy is exemplified in the creation of relaxing VR environments and dynamic avatars, which, when combined with the nuanced conversational abilities of LLMs, offer a novel and potentially transformative approach to mental-health support. However, it is essential to explore the acceptability of such a combination to patients, their willingness to form a therapeutic bond with a VR/AI entity, and the ability of current LLMs to address a diverse array of biopsychosocial issues. Understanding the practicality, safety, and patient receptivity of this innovative psychotherapeutic approach is paramount before its widespread adoption.

At Cedars-Sinai Medical Center in Los Angeles, California, the development of the eXtended-Reality Artificial Intelligence Assistant (XAIA) represents a significant step forward in this domain.[92] This system aims to provide self-directed, AI-facilitated mental-health support within immersive VR settings. On initiating the program, users are immersed in one of nine meticulously crafted nature scenes, ranging from aquatic vistas like tropical beaches to celestial views such as orbiting Earth (see Figure 3.1). The central figure in these scenes is "XAIA," a robot embodying the role of a therapist (see Figure 3.2), offering a unique interaction experience, as showcased in a video available at https://virtualmedicine.org/maia/paper/video. The technical architecture supporting this interaction is robust and privacy-conscious (see Figure 3.3). Audio inputs from the user are securely transmitted to a HIPAA-compliant server, where

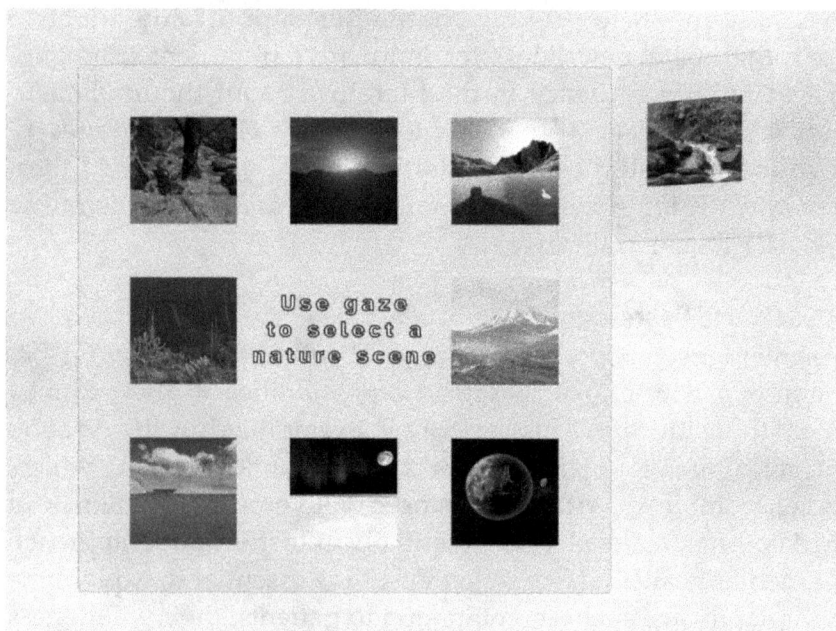

FIGURE 3.1 Nine virtual reality environments for participants' conversation with XAIA. The scenes include a tropical beach, glacial lake, coral reef, desert sunrise, snowy mountain, forest, floating above the clouds, and orbiting Earth.

they are converted to text using advanced speech-to-text AI. The resultant text is processed by GPT-4 to formulate responses, which are then vocalized using a text-to-speech AI characterized by a soothing, reassuring tone. This seamless integration of technologies ensures an engaging and interactive conversation

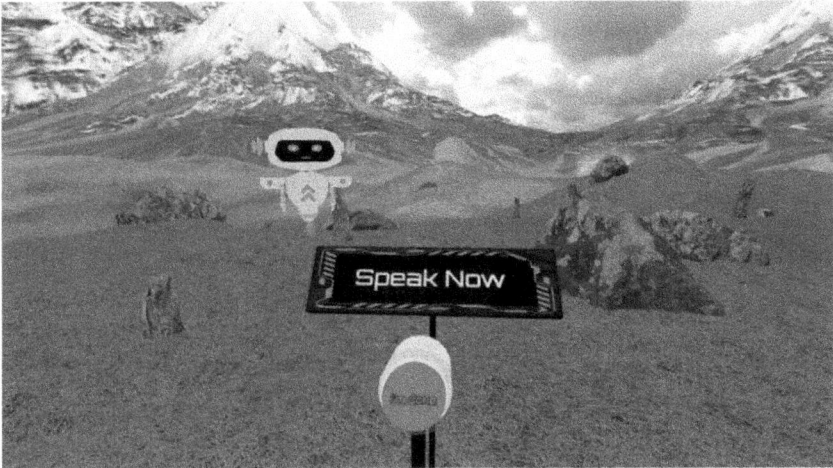

FIGURE 3.2 Actual scene of participants conversing with XAIA. When a participant is done speaking, he/she just needs to look at the green button for a few seconds to allow XAIA to start talking.

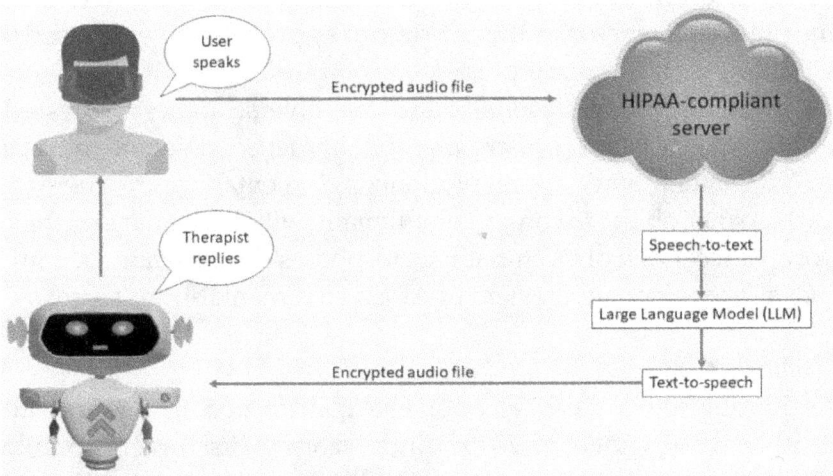

FIGURE 3.3 The data transmission framework of XAIA.

with XAIA, culminating in a session summary that enhances the therapeutic experience.

To ensure the authenticity and effectiveness of the AI therapist, we collaborated with experienced psychotherapists and psychiatrists. This partnership was crucial in establishing system prompts that direct GPT-4 to emulate the empathetic, non-judgmental, and supportive nature of a skilled human therapist. The authenticity of the interaction was further refined using scripts from simulated therapy sessions, thereby aligning the AI's responses with the style and rhythm of professional therapeutic dialogue.

The study involved adult participants with mild to moderate depression or anxiety, as indicated by PHQ-9 of 5–19 or GAD-7 of 5–14. Participants engaged in a 30-minute session with XAIA, followed by a comprehensive 45-minute debriefing interview to glean in-depth insights into their experience. Thematic analysis of these interviews revealed a wide spectrum of therapy topics, reflecting the diverse biopsychosocial challenges faced by the participants. Remarkably, participants often personified the avatar, XAIA, expressing raw emotions and perceiving empathic responses from it. The overall perception of the program was overwhelmingly positive, with many participants highlighting the ease of use, XAIA's approachability, and the empowering nature of the experience. While some participants showed a preference for traditional human therapists, all acknowledged the potential benefits of this AI-driven approach and expressed a willingness to recommend it.

The enthusiastic response and the diverse topics addressed during the sessions underscore the immense potential of this AI-VR integration in revolutionizing mental-health therapy. Participants' ability to connect emotionally with the avatar and their positive reception of its empathetic responses demonstrate a significant advancement in the field of AI-assisted mental-health care.

Alcohol Use Disorder

As highlighted earlier, alcohol use contributed to 5.3% of all deaths worldwide in 2019, underscoring its severe public health consequences. In the United States alone, AUD and alcohol-associated liver disease affect a significant portion of the population, with the prevalence of 10.6% and 4.8% respectively. Although pharmacological interventions such as naltrexone, acamprosate, and baclofen have been instrumental in managing cravings, various psychotherapeutic approaches have proven effective in mitigating the symptoms associated with AUD. Among these, motivational interviewing and CBT stand out as primary treatment modalities. However, there is a substantial unmet need in the provision of CBT and motivational interviewing. Furthermore, stigma, arising from societal misconceptions, stereotypes, and negative attitudes toward those struggling with SUDs, acts as a barrier to seeking treatment for SUD. Many individuals with SUD delay or avoid treatment due to fear of judgment. The perceived stigma from healthcare providers or peers in the treatment group may hinder the effectiveness of interventions.

Given the success of XAIA in delivering CBT for patients with anxiety and depression, we planned to adapt and extend its capabilities to address AUD. To this end, we have integrated motivational interviewing techniques into XAIA, aiming to evaluate its feasibility, safety, and acceptability in the context of VR/ AI therapy for AUD. We engaged the expertise of an addiction medicine specialist and a psychologist with extensive experience in motivational interviewing. These professionals served as standard patients, offering feedback to refine XAIA's updated functionality. Finally, XAIA with motivational interviewing skills in addition to CBT, with no judgmental feedback found in the testing period was generated.

This study enrolls adult patients with alcohol-related cirrhosis, monitored in either inpatient or outpatient settings. Criteria for exclusion include a history of seizure and hepatic encephalopathy grade ≥2, to ensure the safety and appropriateness of the intervention for participants. While the overall study design was consistent with the one previously implemented for anxiety and depression, with 30-minute interactions with XAIA now encompassing both CBT and motivational interviewing, followed by a 45-minute semi-structured interview, we have also incorporated additional questionnaires. These questionnaires are designed to evaluate the usability of XAIA in this new context, providing critical insights into its application in treating alcohol use or preventing relapse.

As the study is currently in the patient enrollment phase, data and results will be forthcoming upon completion and publication. This expansion of XAIA's scope to include nonjudgmental mental-health support for alcohol-related cirrhosis represents a significant advancement in the field of AI-assisted therapy. Through this innovative approach, we aim to not only broaden the therapeutic applications of AI in healthcare but also to offer a novel, engaging, and effective treatment option for individuals grappling with the challenges of SUDs.

Introduction of Generative Reality

The integration of mixed reality, notably through Apple's Vision Pro, heralds a revolutionary approach to the delivery of psychological therapy.[93] This innovative technology blurs the lines between the physical and digital realms, creating an immersive experience that grounds patients in familiar environments while augmenting them with virtual elements. Unlike traditional VR, which secludes users from their real-world surroundings, mixed reality (MR), or computer spacing, maintains this crucial connection, enhancing both comfort and safety during therapeutic sessions.

A pivotal aspect of mental-health treatment is the recognition of facial expressions. The improved capability of facial expression recognition in MR, particularly in combination with AI-enabled CAs, holds immense promise for treating mental-health disorders. This approach offers personalized treatment and potentially enhanced therapeutic outcomes. Recent advancements in this field include the development of lightweight convolutional neural networks like MobileNet V2, capable of detecting emotions within VR settings.[94] Among the leading VR/MR devices, the Apple Vision Pro stands out for its superior facial emotion recognition, allowing the system to discern subtle emotional cues in real time and dynamically tailor treatment interventions.

Another significant advantage of Apple's Vision Pro is its enhanced realism. High-definition rendering elevates the realism of the therapeutic environment, potentially improving the effectiveness of mental-health support. For instance, in exposure therapy, therapists can use Vision Pro to simulate real-life scenarios in a controlled yet authentic setting, surpassing the capabilities of traditional VR. This advancement deepens user immersion in detailed and expansive virtual environments, making therapy sessions more realistic and relatable.

Standing on the foundation of the previous version of XAIA, we developed a new version of XAIA to be a computer spacing app launching on the Apple Vision Pro. XAIA embodies the concept of "Generated Reality" (GR), where AI determines the context of the discussion based on the user's verbal input and generates a therapeutic reality that enhances the emotional impact of therapy (see Figure 3.4). GR employs symbolic imagery, 3D objects, creative particle effects, colors validated through psychometrics, and original music composed to evoke specific emotional responses and dynamic environmental

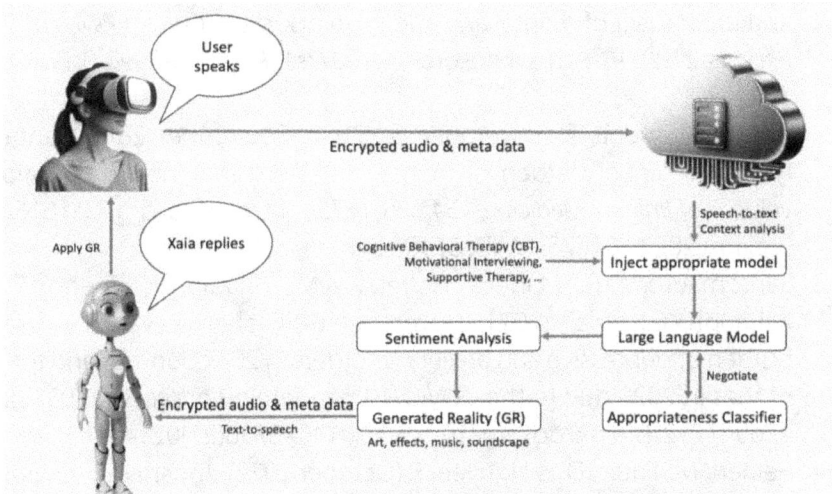

FIGURE 3.4 XAIA data pipeline.
Source: The figure was adapted from a recent publication of the team on *NPJ Digital Medicine.*

interactions. To facilitate GR on the Vision Pro, we have created a comprehensive library of contexts and effects designed to subtly influence the subconscious.

XAIA's functionalities extend to personalized therapeutic support and AI-tailored meditation, ensuring all user data are stored in compliance with HIPAA regulations. GR's ability to analyze, adapt, and respond to user inputs in real time fosters a deeper connection and engagement with the virtual world. The combination of graphical effects and carefully chosen music enhances the user experience in various psychotherapies, such as exposure therapy for anxiety and phobia treatment.

For further information on this groundbreaking integration of technology and therapy, additional details can be found on the associated webpage (https://www.xaia.health/). Through XAIA and the Apple Vision Pro, we are poised to redefine the landscape of mental-health treatment, offering more immersive, personalized, and effective therapeutic experiences.

References

1 Rehm, J., & Shield, K.D. (2019, February 7). Global burden of disease and the impact of mental and addictive disorders. *Current Psychiatry Reports, 21*(2), 10. https://doi.org/10.1007/s11920-019-0997-0. PMID: 30729322.

2 Arias, D., Saxena, S., & Verguet, S. (2022, September 28). Quantifying the global burden of mental disorders and their economic value. *eClinical Medicine, 54*, 101675. https://doi.org/10.1016/j.eclinm.2022.101675. PMID: 36193171.

3 Santomauro, D.F., Mantilla Herrera, A.M., Shadid, J., Zheng, P., Asbaugh, C., et al. (2021, November 6). Global prevalence and burden of depressive and anxiety disorders in 204 countries and territories in 2020 due to the COVID-19 pandemic. *Lancet, 398*(10312), 1700–1712. https://doi.org/10.1016/S0140–6736(21)02143-7

4 Reinert, M., Fritze, D., & Nguyen, T. (October 2022). *The state of mental health in America 2023*. Alexandria, VA: Mental Health America.

5 National Institute of Mental Health. (n.d.). Statistics. Retrieved from https://www.nimh.nih.gov/health/statistics/mental-illness

6 Reinert, M., Fritze, D., & Nguyen, T. (October 2022). *The state of mental health in America 2023*. Alexandria, VA: Mental Health America.

7 Cleare, A., Pariante, C.M., Young, A.H., Anderson, I.M., Christmas, D., et al. (May, 2015). Evidence-based guidelines for treating depressive disorders with antidepressants: A revision of the 2008 British Association for psychopharmacology guidelines. *Journal of Psychopharmacology, 29*(5), 459–525. PMID 25969470.

8 Hofmann, S.G., Asnaani, A., Vonk, I.J., Sawyer, A.T., & Fang, A. (2012, October 1). The efficacy of cognitive behavioral therapy: A review of meta-analyses. *Cognitive Therapy Research, 36*(5), 427–440. https://doi.org/10.1007/s10608-012-9476-1. PMID: 23459093.

9 Nakao, M., Shirotsuki, K., & Sugaya, N. (2021, October 3). Cognitive behavioral therapy for management of mental health and stress-related disorders: Recent advances in techniques and technologies. *Biopsychosocial Medicine, 15*(1), 16. https://doi.org/10.1186/s13030-021-00219-w. PMID: 34602086.

10 Hoffman, S.G., & Smits, J.A. (2008, April). Cognitive-behavioral therapy for adult anxiety disorders: A meta-analysis of randomized placebo-controlled trials. *Journal of Clinical Psychiatry, 69*(4), 621–632. https://doi.org/10.4088/jcp.v69n0415. PMID: 18363421.

11 Van Straten, A., Geraedts, A., Verdonck-de Leeuw, I., Andersson, G., & Cuijpers, P. (2010, July). Psychological treatment of depressive symptoms in patients with medical disorders: A meta-analysis. *Journal of Psychosomatic Research, 69*(1), 23–32. https://doi.org/10.1016/j.jpsychores.2010.01.019. PMID: 20630260; Beltman, M.W., Voshaar, R.C., & Speckens, A.E. (2010, July). Cognitive-behavioural therapy for depression in people with a somatic disease: Meta-analysis of randomized controlled trials. *British Journal of Psychiatry, 197*(1), 11–19. https://doi.org/10.1192/bjp.bp.109.054675. PMID: 20592427.

12 Miller, W.R., & Rollnick, S. (2002). *Motivational interviewing: Preparing people for change* (2nd ed.). New York: Guilford Press.

13 Peterson, P.L., Baer, J.S., Wells, E.A., Ginzler, J.A., & Garrett, S.B. (2006, September). Short-term effects of a brief motivational intervention to reduce alcohol and drug risk among homeless adolescents. *Psychology of Addictive Behavior, 20*(3), 254–264. https://doi.org/10.1037/0893-164X.20.3.254. PMID: 16938063.

14 Riper, H., Andersson, G., Hunter, S.B., de Wit, J., Berking, M., & Cuijpers, P. (2014, March). Treatment of comorbid alcohol use

disorders and depression with cognitive-behavioural therapy and motivational interviewing: A meta-analysis. *Addiction, 109*(3), 394–406. https://doi.org/10.1111/add.12441. PMID: 24304463.

15 Cuijpers, P., Dekker, J., Hollon, S.D., & Andersson, G. (2009, September). Adding psychotherapy to pharmacotherapy in the treatment of depressive disorders in adults: A meta-analysis. *Journal of Clinical Psychiatry, 70*(9), 1219–1229. https://doi.org/10.4088/JCP.09r05021. PMID 19818243; Cuijpers, P., van Straten, A., Warmerdam, L., & Andersson, G. (2009). Psychotherapy versus the combination of psychotherapy and pharmacotherapy in the treatment of depression: A meta-analysis. *Depression and Anxiety, 26*(3), 279–288. https://doi.org/10.1002/da.20519. PMID 19031487.

16 Glueckauf, R.L., Pickett, T.C., Ketterson, T.U., Loomis, J.S., & Rozensky, R.H. (2003). Preparation for the delivery of telehealth services: A self-study framework for expansion of practice. *Professional Psychology: Research and Practice, 34*(2), 159–163. https://doi.org/10.1037/0735-7028.34.2.159.

17 Sahin, E., Yavuz Veizi, B.G., & Naharci, M.I. (2024, February). Telemedicine interventions for older adults: A systematic review. *Journal of Telemedicine and Telecare, 30*(2), 305–319. https://doi.org/10.1177/1357633X211058340. PMID: 34825609; Kim, E.H., Gellis, Z.D., Bradway, C.K., & Kenaley, B. (2019, September). Depression care services and telehealth technology use for homebound elderly in the United States. *Aging Mental Health, 23*(8), 1164–1173. https://doi.org/10.1080/13607863.2018.1481925. PMID: 30472881.

18 Brenes, G.A., Ingram, C.W., & Danhauer, S.C. (2011, December). Benefits and challenges of conducting psychotherapy by telephone. *Professional Psychology, Research and Practice, 42*(6), 543–549. https://doi.org/10.1037/a0026135. PMID: 22247588.

19 Swinson, R.P., Fergus, K.D., Cox, G.J., & Wickwire, K. (1995). Efficacy of telephone administered behavioral therapy for panic disorder with agoraphobia. *Behaviour Research and Therapy, 33*(4), 465–469. https://doi.org/10.1016/0005-8067(94)00061-n. PMID: 7755536.

20 Lovell, K., Cox, D., Haddock, G., Jones, C., Raines, D., Garvey, R., Roberts, C., & Hadley, S. (2006). Telephone administered cognitive behaviour therapy for treatment of obsessive compulsive disorder: Randomised controlled non-inferiority trial. *BMJ (Clinical Research ed.), 333*(7574), 883. PMID: 16935946.

21 Brenes, G.A., Miller, M.E., Williamson, J.D., McCall, W.V., Knudson, M., & Stanley, M.A. (2012). A randomized controlled trial of telephone-delivered cognitive-behavioral therapy for late-life anxiety disorders. *American Journal of Geriatric Psychiatry, 20*(8), 707–716. https://doi.org/10.1097/JGP.0b013e318ssccd3e. PMID: 22828172.

22 Mozer, E., Franklin, B., & Rose, J. (2008). Psychotherapeutic intervention by telephone. *Clinical Interventions in Aging, 3*(2), 391–396. https://doi.org/10.2147/cia.s950. PMID: 18686761.

23 Tarp, K., Bojesen, A.B., Mejldal, A., & Nielsen, A.S. (2017). Effectiveness of optional videoconferencing-based treatment of alcohol use disorders: Randomized controlled trial. *JMIR Mental Health, 4*(3), e38. https://doi.org/10.2196/mental.6713. PMID: 28963093.

24 House Resolution No. 6., SUPPORT for Patients and Communities Act, 115th Congress. (2017–2018). Public Law No: 115–271 (10/24/2018).

25 Marcelle, E.T., Nolting, L., Hinshaw, S.P., & Aguilera, A. (2019). Effectiveness of a multimodal digital psychotherapy platform for adult depression: A naturalistic feasibility study. *JMIR mHealth and uHealth, 7*(1), e10948. https://doi.org/10.2196/10948. PMID: 30674448.

26 Reinert, M., Fritze, D., & Nguyen, T. (October 2022). *The state of mental health in America 2023*. Alexandria, VA: Mental Health America.

27 Hockenberry, J.M., Joski, P., Yarbrough, C., & Druss, B.G. (2019). Trends in treatment and spending for patients receiving outpatient treatment of depression in the United States, 1998–2015. *JAMA Psychiatry, 76*(8), 810–817. https://doi.org/10.1001/jamapsychiatry.2019.063. PMID: 31017627.

28 Walker, E.R., Cummings, J.R., Hockenberry, J.M., & Druss, B.G. (2015). Insurance status, use of mental health services, and unmet need for mental health care in the United States. *Psychiatric Services* (Washington, D.C.), *66*(6), 578–584. https://doi.org/10.1176/appi.ps.201400248. PMID: 25726980; Gulliver, A., Griffiths, K.M., & Christensen, H. (2010). Perceived barriers and facilitators to mental health help-seeking in young people: A systematic review. *BMC Psychiatry, 10*, 113. https://doi.org/10.1186/1471-244X-10–113. PMID: 21192795; Toso Salman, J., Wald, M., Hoffman, L., Brody, H., & Feliz, L. (2022). Assessing barriers to engagement in a community mental health center using the Psychosocial Assessment Tool (PAT). *Psychological Services*. https://doi.org/10.1037/ser0000647. Advance online publication. PMID: 35311342.

29 Walker, E.R., Cummings, J.R., Hockenberry, J.M., & Druss, B.G. (2015). Insurance status, use of mental health services, and unmet need for mental health care in the United States. *Psychiatric Services* (Washington, D.C.), *66*(6), 578–584. https://doi.org/10.1176/appi. ps.201400248. PMID: 25726980.

30 Dinh, H.Q., Walker, N., Hodges, L.F., Song, C., & Kobayashi, A. (1999). Evaluating the importance of multi-sensory input on memory and the sense of presence in virtual environments. *Proceedings IEEE Virtual Reality Houston, TX*, 222–228. https://doi.org/10.1109/ VR.1999.756955

31 Slater, M. (2009). Place illusion and plausibility can lead to real-istic behaviour in immersive virtual environments. *Philosophical Transactions of the Royal Society of London. Series B., Biological Sciences, 364*(1535), 3549–3557. https://doi.org/10.1098/rstb.2009.0138. PMID: 19884149; Li, S., Gu, X., Yi, K., Yang, Y, Wang, G., & Manocha, D. (2022). Self-illusion: A study on cognition of role-playing in immersive virtual environments. *IEEE Transactions on Visualization and Computer Graphics, 28*(8), 3035–3049. https://doi.org/10.1109/ TVCG.2020.3044563. PMID: 33315568.

32 Freeman, D., Reeve, S., Robinson, A., Ehlers, A., Clark, D., Spanlang, B., & Slater, M. (2017). Virtual reality in the assessment, understanding, and treatment of mental health disorders. *Psychological Medicine, 47*(14), 2393–2400. https://doi.org/10.1017/S000-3329171700040X. PMID: 28325167.

33 Wienrich, C., Döllinger, N., & Hein, R. (2021). Behavioral framework of immersive technologies (BehaveFIT), How and why virtual reality can support behavioral change processes. *Frontiers in Virtual Reality, 2*, 627194. https://doi.org/10.3389/frvir.2021.627194

34 Jingili, N., Oyelere, S.S., Nyström, M.B.T., & Anyshchenko, L. (2023). A systematic review on the efficacy of virtual reality and gamification interventions for managing anxiety and depres-sion. *Frontiers in Digital Health, 5*, 1239435. https://doi.org/10.3389/ fdgth.2023.1239435. PMID: 38026832.

35 Carlin, A.S., Hoffman, H.G., & Weghorst, S. (1997). Virtual reality and tactile augmentation in the treatment of spider phobia: A case report. *Behaviour Research and Therapy, 35*(2), 153–158. https://doi. org/10.1016/s0005-7967(96)00085-x. PMID: 9046678.

36 Hodges, L.F., Kooper, R., Meyer, T.C., Rothbaum, B.O., Opdyke, D., de Graff, J.J., Williford, J.S., & North, M.M. (1995, July). Virtual environments for treating the fear of heights. *Computer, 28*(7), 27–34. https://doi.org/10.1109/2.391038

37 Rothbaum, B.O., Hodges, L., Watson, B.A., Kessler, C.D., & Opdyke, D. (1996). Virtual reality exposure therapy in the treatment of fear of flying: A case report. *Behaviour Research and Therapy, 34*(5–6), 477–481. https://doi.org/10.1016/0005-7967(96)00007-1. PMID: 8687369.

38 Botella, C., Baños, R.M., Perpiña, C., Villa, H., Alcañiz, M., & Rey, A. (1998). Virtual reality treatment of claustrophobia: A case report. *Behaviour Research and Therapy, 36*(2), 129–146. https://doi.org/10.1016/s0005-7967(97)10006-7. PMID: 9613029.

39 Difede, J., & Hoffman, H.G., (2002). Virtual reality exposure therapy for World Trade Center port-traumatic stress disorder: A case report. *Cyberpsychology & Behavior: The Impact of the Internet, Multimedia and Virtual Reality on Behavior and Society, 5*(6), 529–535. https://doi.org/10.1089/109493102321018169. PMID: 12556115; Difede, J., Cukor, J., Jayasinghe, N., Patt, I, Jedel, S., Spielman, L., Giosan, C., & Hoffman, H.G. (2007). Virtual reality exposure therapy for the treatment of posttraumatic stress disorder following September 11, 2001. *Journal of Clinical Psychiatry, 68*(11), 1639–1647. PMID: 18052556.

40 Rothbaum, B.O., Hodges, L., Anderson, P.L., Price, L., & Smith, S. (2002). Twelve-month follow-up of virtual reality and standard exposure therapies for the fear of flying. *Journal of Consulting and Clinical Psychology, 70*(2), 428–432. https://doi.org/10.1037//0022-006x.70.2.428. PMID: 11952201; Wiederhold, B.K., & Wiederhold, M.D. (2003). Three-year follow-up for virtual reality exposure for fear of flying. *Cyberpsychology & Behavior: The Impact of the Internet, Multimedia, and Virtual Reality on Behavior and Society, 6*(4), 441–445. https://doi.org/10.1089/109493103322278844. PMID: 14511458.

41 Anderson, P.L., Price, M., Edwards, S.M., Obasaju, M.A., Schmertz, S.K., Zimand, E., & Calamaras, M.R. (2013). Virtual reality exposure therapy for social anxiety disorder: A randomized controlled trial. *Journal of Consulting and Clinical Psychology, 81*(5), 751–760. https://doi.org/10.1037/a0033559. PMID: 23796315; Bouchard, S., Dumoulin, S., Robillard, G., Guitard, T., Klinger, É., Forget, H.,

Loranger, C., & Roucaut, F.X. (2017). Virtual reality compared with in vivo exposure in the treatment of social anxiety disorder: A three-arm randomized controlled trial. *British Journal of Psychiatry, 210*(4), 276–283. https://doi.org/10.1192/bjp.bp.116.184234. PMID: 27979818.

42 Gorini, A., Pallavicini, F., Algeri, D., Repetto, C., Gaggioli, A., & Riva, G. (2010). Virtual reality in the treatment of generalized anxiety disorders. *Studies in Health Technology and Informatics, 154*, 39–43. PMID: 20543266.

43 Cardos, R.A.I., David, O.A., & David, D.O. (2017). Virtual reality exposure therapy in flight anxiety: A quantitative meta-analysis. *Computers in Human Behavior, 72*, 371–380. https://doi.org/10.1016/j.chb.2017.03.007

44 García-Palacios, A., Botella, C., Hoffman, H., & Fabregat, S. (2007). Comparing acceptance and refusal rates of virtual reality exposure vs. in vivo exposure by patients with specific phobias. *Cyberpsychology & Behavior: The Impact of the Internet, Multimedia, and Virtual Reality on Behavior and Society, 10*(5), 722–724. https://doi.org/10.1089/cpb.2007.9962. PMID: 17927544.

45 Fodor, L.A., Cotet, C.D., Cuijpers, P., Szamoskozi, S., David, D., & Cristea, I.A. (2018). The effectiveness of virtual-reality based interventions for symptoms of anxiety and depression: A meta-analysis. *Scientific Reports, 8*(1), 10323. https://doi.org/10.1038/s41598-018-28113-6. PMID: 29985400.

46 Van Loenen, I., Scholten, W., Muntingh, A., Smit, J., & Batelaan, N. (2002). The effectiveness of virtual-reality based exposure-based cognitive behavioral therapy for severe anxiety disorders, obsessive-compulsive disorder, and posttraumatic stress disorder: Meta-analysis. *Journal of Medical Internet Research, 24*(2), 326736. https://doi.org/10.2196/26736. PMID: 35142632.

47 Opris, D., Pintea, S., García-Palacios, A., Botella, C., Szamosközi, S., & David, D. (2012). Virtual reality exposure therapy in anxiety disorders: A quantitative meta-analysis. *Depression and Anxiety, 29*(2), 85–93. https://doi.org/10.1002/da.20910. PMID: 22065564.

48 Wu, J., Sun, Y., Zhang, G., Zhou, Z., & Ren, Z. (2021). Virtual reality-assisted cognitive behavioral therapy for anxiety disorders: A systematic review and meta-analysis. *Frontiers in Psychiatry, 12*, 575094. https://doi.org/10.3389/fpsyt.2021.575094. PMID: 34366904.

49 Van Loenen, I., Scholten, W., Muntingh, A., Smit, J., & Batelaan, N. (2002). The effectiveness of virtual-reality based exposure-based cognitive behavioral therapy for severe anxiety disorders, obsessive-compulsive disorder, and posttraumatic stress disorder: Meta-analysis. *Journal of Medical Internet Research, 24*(2), 326736. https://doi.org/10.2196/26736. PMID: 35142632.

50 Dangare, M., & Yadav, V. (2023). Gaming on an immersive virtual reality platform to ameliorate the level of anxiety in patients under-going congenital heart disease. *Cureus, 15*(12), 350694. https://doi.org/10.7759/cureus.50694. PMID: 38234943.

51 Rizzo, A., Roy, M.J., Hartholt, A., Costanzo, M. Highland, K.B., Jovanovic, T., Norrholm, S.D., Reist, C., Rothbaum, B., & Difede, J. (2017). In S.V. Bowles & P.T. Bartone (Eds.), *Handbook of Military Psychology*, pp. 453–471. Cham: Springer International.

52 Rizzo, A., & Shilling, R. (2017). Clinical virtual reality tools to advance the prevention, assessment, and treatment of PTSD. *European Journal of Psychotraumatology, 8*(sup5), 1414560. https://doi.org/10.1080/20008198.2017.1414560. PMID: 29372007.

53 Beck, J.G., Palyo, S.A., Winer, E.H., Schwagler, B.E., & Ang, E.J. (2007). Virtual reality exposure therapy for PTSD symptoms after a road accident: An uncontrolled case series. *Behavior Therapy, 38*(1), 39–48. https://doi.org/10.1016/j.beth.2006.04.001. PMID: 17292693.

54 Knaust, T., Felnhofer, A., Kothgassner, O.D., Höllmer, H., Gorzka, R.J., & Schulz, H. (2020). Virtual trauma interventions for the treatment of post-traumatic stress disorders: A scoping review. *Frontiers in Psychology, 11*, 562506. https://doi.org/10.3389/fpsyg.2020.562506. PMID: 33281664; Ménélas, B.J., Haidon, C., Ecrepont, A., & Girard, B. (2018). Use of virtual reality technologies as an action-cue exposure therapy for truck drivers suffering from post-traumatic stress disorder. *Entertainment Computing, 24*, 1–9.

55 Rothbaum, B.O., Hodges, L., Alarcon, R., Ready, D., Shahar, F., Graap, K., Pair, J., Hebert, P., Gotz, D., wills, B., & Baltzell, D. (1999). Virtual reality exposure therapy for PTSD Vietnam veterans: A case study. *Journal of Traumatic Stress, 12*(2), 263–271. https://doi.org/10.1023/A:1024772308758. PMID: 10378165; Gamito, P., Oliveira, J., Morais, D., Saraiva, T., Rosa, P.J., Leal, A., Pacheco, J., Ribeiro, C., Dias Neto, D., & Pablo, C. (2007). War PTSD: A VR pretrial case study. *Annual Review of Cybertherapy and Telemedicine, 5*, 191–198.

56 Wood, D.P., Roy, M.J., Wiederhold, B.K., & Wiederhold, M.D. (2021). Combat-related posttraumatic stress disorder: A case report of virtual reality graded exposure therapy with physiological monitoring in a US Navy officer and a US Army officer. *Cureus, 13*(11), e19604. https://doi.org/10.7759/cureus.19604. PMID: 34926073.

57 Difede, J., & Hoffman, H.G., (2002). Virtual reality exposure therapy for World Trade Center port-traumatic stress disorder: A case report. *Cyberpsychology & Behavior: The Impact of the Internet, Multimedia and Virtual Reality on Behavior and Society, 5*(6), 529–535. https://doi.org/10.1089/109493102321018169. PMID: 12556115.

58 Reger, G.M., Koenen-Woods, P., Zetocha, K., Smolenski, D.J., Holloway, K.M., Rothbaum, B.O., Difede, J., Rizzo, A.A., Edwards-Stewart, A., Skopp, N.A., Mishkind, M., Reger, M.A., & Gahm, G.A. (2016). Randomized controlled trial of prolonged exposure using imaginal exposure vs. virtual reality exposure in active-duty soldiers with deployment-related posttraumatic stress disorder (PTSD). *Journal of Consulting and Clinical Psychology, 84*(11), 946–959. https://doi.org/10.1037/ccp0000134. PMID: 27606699.

59 Heo, S., & Park, J.H. (2022) Effects of virtual reality-based graded exposure therapy on PTSD symptoms: A systematic review and meta-analysis. *International Journal of Environmental Research and Public Health, 19*(23), 15911. https://doi.org/10.3390/ijerph192315911. PMID: 36497989.

60 Falconer, C.J., Rovira, A., King, J.A., Gilbert, P., Antley, A., Fearon, P., Ralph, N., Slater, M., & Brewin, C.R. (2016). Embodying self-compassion within virtual reality and its effects on patients with depression. *BJPsych open, 2*(1), 74–80. https://doi.org/10.1192/bjpo.bp.115.002147. PMID: 27703757.

61 Dehn, L.B., Kater, L., Piefke, M., Botsch, M., Driessen, M., &T. Beblo, T. (2018). Training in a comprehensive everyday-like virtual reality environment compared to computerized cognitive training for patients with depression. *Computers in Human Behavior, 79*, 40–52. Retrieved from https://www.sciencedirect.com/science/article/abs/pii/S0747563217305927

62 Suwanjatuporn, A., & Chintakovid, T. (2019). Using a virtual reality system to improve quality of life of the elderly people with depression. *IEEE International Conference on Consumer Electronics—Asia*, pp. 153–156. https://doi.org/10.1109/ICCE-Asia46551.2019.8941607

63 Stamou, G., García-Palacios, A., & Botella, C. (2019, December). The combination of cognitive-behavioural therapy with virtual reality for the treatment of post-natal depression. *OzCHI'19: Proceedings of the 31st Australian Conference on Human-Computer-Interaction.*

64 Shah, L.B., Torres, S., Kannusamy, P., Chng, C.M., He, H.G., & Klainin-Yobas, P. (2014). Efficacy of the virtual reality-based stress management program on stress-related variables in people with mood disorders: The feasibility study. *Archives of Psychiatric Nursing, 29*(1), 6–13. https://doi.org/10.1016/j.apnu.2014.09.003. PMID: 25634868.

65 Lee, N.Y., Lee, D.K., & Song, H.S. (2015). Effect of virtual reality dance exercise on the balance, activities of daily living, and depressive disorder status of Parkinson's disease patients. *Journal of Physical Therapy Science, 27*(1), 145–147. https://doi.org/10.1589/jpts.27.145. PMID: 25642060.

66 Ferguson, S.G., & Shiffman, S. (2009). The relevance and treatment of cue-induced cravings in tobacco dependence. *Journal of Substance Abuse Treatment, 36*(3), 235–243. https://doi.org/10.1016/j.jsat.2008.06.005. PMID: 18715743.

67 Perry, J.L., Joseph, J.E., Jiang, Y., Zimmerman, R.S., Kelly, T.H., Darna, M., Huettl, P., Dwoskin, L.P., & Bardo, M.T. (2011). Prefrontal cortex and drug abuse vulnerability: Translation to prevention and treatment interventions. *Brain Research Reviews, 65*(2), 124–149. https://doi.org/10.1016/j.brainresrev.2010.09.001. PMID: 20837060.

68 Girard, B., Turcotte, V., Bouchard, S., & Girard, B. (2009). Crushing virtual cigarettes reduced tobacco addiction and treatment discontinuation. *Cyberpsychology & Behavior: The Impact of the Internet, Multimedia, and Virtual Reality on Behavior and Society, 12*(5), 477–483. https://doi.org/10.1089/cpb.2009.0118. PMID: 19817561.

69 Hone-Blanchet, A., Wensing, T., & Fecteau, S. (2014). The use of virtual reality in craving assessment and cue-exposure therapy in substance use disorders. *Frontiers in Human Neuroscience, 8*, 844. https://doi.org/10.3389/fnhum.2014.00844. PMID: 25368571.

70 Drummond, D.C., Cooper, T., & Glautier, S.P. (1990). Conditioned learning in alcohol dependence: Implications for cue exposure treatment. *British Journal of Addiction, 85*(6), 725–743. https://doi.org/10.1111/j.1360-0443.1990.tb01685.x. PMID: 2198966.

71 Lee, J.H., Ku, J., Kim, K., Kim, B., Kim, I.Y., Yang, B.H., Kim, S.H., Wiederhold, B.K., Wiederhold, M.D., Park, D.W., Lim, Y., & Kim, S.I. (2003). Experimental application of virtual reality for nicotine craving through cue exposure. *Cyberpsychology & Behavior: The Impact of the Internet, Multimedia, and Virtual Reality on Behavior and Society, 6*(3), 275–280. https://doi.org/10.1089.109493103322011560. PMID: 12855083; Lee, J.H., Lim, Y., Wiederhold, B.K., & Graham, S.J. (2005). A functional magnetic resonance imaging (fMRI) study of cue-induced smoking craving in virtual environments. *Applied Psychophysiology and Biofeedback, 30*(3), 195–204. https://doi.org/10.1007/s10484-005-6377-z. PMID: 16167185.

72 Pericot-Valverde, I., García-Rodríguez, O., Gutierrez-Maldonado, J., Ferrer-García, M., & Secades-Villa, R. (2011). Evolution of smoking urge during exposure through virtual reality. *Studies in Health Technology and Informatics, 167*, 74–79. PMID: 21685645.

73 Traylor, A.C., Bordnick, P.S., & Carter, B.L. (2009). Using virtual reality to assess young adult smokers' attention to cues. *Cyberpsychology & Behavior: The Impact of the Internet, Multimedia, and Virtual Reality on Behavior and Society, 12*(4), 373–378. https://doi.org/10.1089/cpb.2009.0070. PMID: 19630582.

74 Ryan, J.J., Kreiner, D.S., Chapman, M.D., & Stark-Wroblewski, K. (2010). Virtual reality cues for binge drinking in college students. *Cyberpsychology, Behavior, and Social Networking, 13*(2), 159–162. https://doi.org/10.1089/cyber.2009.0211. PMID: 20528271.

75 Lee, S.H., Han, D.H., Oh, S., Lyoo, I.K., Lee, Y.S., Renshaw, P.F., & Lukas, S.E. (2009). Quantitative electroencephalographic (qEEG) correlates of craving during virtual reality therapy in alcohol-dependent patients. *Pharmacology, Biochemistry, and Behavior, 91*(3), 393–397. https://doi.org/10.1016/j.pbb.2008.08.014. PMID: 18771681.

76 Zhang, J., Chen, M., Yan, J., Wang, C., Deng, H., Wang, J., Gu, J., Wang, D., Li, W., & Wang, C. (2023). Effects of virtual reality-based cue exposure therapy on craving and physiological responses in alcohol-dependent patients: A randomized controlled trial. *BMC Psychiatry, 23*(1), 951. https://doi.org/10.1186/s12888-023-05426-z. PMID: 38110900.

77 Chiang, C.H., Huang, C.M., Sheu, J.J., Liao, J.Y., Hus, H.P., Wang, S.W., & Guo, J.L. (2021). Examining the effectiveness of 3D virtual reality training on problem-solving, self-efficacy, and teamwork among

inexperienced volunteers helping with drug use prevention: Randomized controlled trial. *Journal of Medical Internet Research, 23*(11), e29862. https://doi.org/10.2196/29862. PMID: 34726606.

78 Peixoto, B., Pinto, R.D., Melo, M., Cabral, L., & Bessa, M. (2021). Immersive virtual reality for foreign language education: A PRISMA systematic review. *IEEE Access, 9*, 48952–48962. https://doi.org/10.1109/ACCESS.2021.3068858

79 Milne-Ives, M., de Cock, C., Lim, E., Shehadeh, M.H., de Pennington, N., Mole, G., Normando, E., & Meinert, E. (2020). The effectiveness of artificial intelligence conversational agents in health care: Systemic review. *Journal of Medical Internet Research, 22*(10), e20346. https://doi.org/10.2196/20346. PMID: 33090118.

80 Koutsouleris, N., Hauser, T.U., Skvortsova, V., & De Choudhury, M. (2022). From promise to practice: Towards the realization of AI-informed mental health care. *Lancet. Digital Health, 4*(11), e829–e840. https://doi.org/10.1016.S2589-7500(22)00153-4. PMID: 36229346.

81 Yeo, Y.H., Samaan, J.S., Ng, W.., Ting, P.S., Trivedi, H., Vipani, A., Ayoub, W., Yang, J.D., Liran, O., Spiegel, B., & Kuo, A. (2023). Assessing the performance of ChatGPT in answering questions regarding cirrhosis and hepatocellular carcinoma. *Clinical and Molecular Hepatology, 29*(3), 721–732. https://doi.org/10.3350/cmn.2023.0089. PMID: 36946005; Samaan, J.S., Yeo, Y.H., Rajeev, N., Hawley, L., Abel, S., Ng, W.H., Srinivasan, N., Park, J., Burch, M., Watson, R., Liran, O., & Samakar, K. (2023). Assessing the accuracy of responses by the language model ChatGPT to questions regarding bariatric surgery. *Obesity Surgery, 33*(6), 1790–1796. https://doi.org/10.1007/s11695-023-06603-5. PMID: 37106269.

82 Achiam, J., et al. (2023). GPT-4 technical report. Cornell University Computer Science. Retrieved from https://doi.org/10.48550/arXiv.2303.08774

83 Abd-Alrazaq, A.A., Rababeh, A., Alajlani, M., Bewick, B.M., & Househ, M. (2020). Effectiveness and safety of using chatbots to improve mental health: Systematic review and meta-analysis. *Journal of Medical Internet Research, 22*(7), e16021. https://doi.org/10.2196/16021. PMID: 32673216.

84 Li, H., Zhang, R., Lee, Y.C., Kraut, R.E., & Mohr, D.C. (2023). Systematic review and meta-analysis of AI-based conversational agents for promoting mental health and well-being. *NPJ Digital Medicine, 6*(1), 236. https://doi.org/10.1038/s4746-023-00979-5. PMID: 38114588.

85 Sedotto, R.N.M., Edwards, A.E., Duplin, P.L., & King, D.K. (2024). Engagement with mHealth alcohol interventions: User perspectives on an app or chatbot-delivered program to reduce drinking. *Healthcare (Basel, Switzerland), 12*(1), 101. https://doi.org/10.3390/healthcare12010101. PMID: 38201007.

86 Fulmer, R., Joerin, A., Gentile, B., Lakerink, L., & Rauws, M. (2018). Using psychological artificial intelligence (Tess) to relieve symptoms of depression and anxiety: Randomized controlled trial. *JMIR Mental Health, 5*(4), e64. https://doi.org/10.2196/mental.9782. PMID: 30545815.

87 Prochaska, J.J., Vogel, E.A., Chieng, A., Kendra, M., Baiocchi, M., Pajarito, S., & Robinson, A. (2021). A therapeutic relational agent for reducing problematic substance use (Woebot), Development and usability study. *Journal of Medical Internet Research, 23*(3), e24850. https://doi.org/10.2196/24850. PMID: 33755028.

88 Prochaska, J.J., Vogel, E.A., Chieng, A., Baiocchi, M., Maglalang, D.D., Pajarito, S., Weingardt, K.R., Darcy, A., & Robinson, A. (2021). A randomized controlled trial of a therapeutic relational agent for reducing substance misuse during the COVID-19 pandemic. *Drug and Alcohol Dependence, 227*, 108986. https://doi.org/10.1016/j.drugalcdep.2021.108986. PMID: 34507061; Chiauzzi, E., Williams, A., Mariano, T.Y., Pajarito, S., Robinson, A., Kirvin-Quamme, A., & Forman-Hoffman, V. (2024). Demographic and clinical characteristics associated with anxiety and depressive symptom outcomes in users of a digital mental health intervention incorporating a relational agent. *BMC Psychiatry, 24*, 79. https://doi.org/10.1186/s12888-024-05532-6. PMID: 38291369.

89 Lee, A.J., Schuelke, M.J., Hunt, D.M., Miller, J.P., Areán, P.A., & Cheng, A.L. (2022). Digital mental health intervention plus usual care compared with usual care only and usual care plus in-person psychological counseling for orthopedic patients with symptoms of depression or anxiety: Cohort study. *JMIR Formative Research, 6*(5), e36203. https://doi.org/10.2196/36203. PMID: 35507387.

90 Trappey, A.J.C., Trappey, C.V., Chao, M.-H., Hong, N.-J., & Wu, C.-T. (2022). A VR-enabled chatbot supporting design and manufacturing of large and complex power transformers. *Electronics, 11*(1), 87. Retrieved from https://doi.org/10.3390/electronics11010087

91 Chow, A.R. (2023, January 27). Why the AI explosion has huge implications for the metaverse. *Time*. Retrieved from https://time.com/6250249/chatgpt-metaverse/

92 Spiegel, B.M.R., Liran, O., Clark, A., et al. (2024). Feasibility of combining spatial computing and AI for mental health support in anxiety and depression. *NPJ Digital Medicine, 7*, 22. https://doi.org/10.1038/s41746-024-01011-0

93 Zhang, Z., Giménez Mateu, L.G., & Fort, J.M. (2023). Apple vision pro: A new horizon in psychological research and therapy. *Frontiers in Psychology, 14*, 1280213. https://doi.org/10.3389/fpsyg.2023.1280213. PMID: 38023044.

94 Zhang, Z., Fort, J.M., & Giménez Mateu, L. (2023). Facial expression recognition in virtual reality environments: Challenges and opportunities. *Frontiers in Psychology, 14*, 1280136. https://doi.org/10.3389/fpsyg.2023.1280136. PMID: 37885738.

4

Virtual Reality in Children and Adolescents with Pain and Palliative-Care Needs

Anna Zanin, Anna Mercante, and Franca Benini

Virtual Reality in Pediatric Pain and Palliative Care

Pain is a common experience in infants and children requiring medical attention.[1] Prevention and treatment of pain in pediatric patients have been repeatedly shown to be inadequate and also less often implemented in comparison to adults, the greater the younger the children are.[2] According to recent definitions, pain is multidimensional in nature, including both sensory (i.e., pain intensity) and emotional correlates (i.e., any negative affect secondary to pain such as distress) associated with actual or potential tissue damage.[3] Pain intensity and pain-related distress (stress, anxiety, fear, frustration) constitutes two essential and unmutual dimensions to consider when defining strategies to manage pain associated with medical interventions.[4] These components are intensely subjective and may sometimes be difficult to distinguish, particularly in nonverbal patients who may be unable to differentiate pain from other unpleasant emotions.[5]

DOI: 10.4324/9781032649771-4

Examinations, procedures, and treatments typical of the healthcare setting represent often an inevitable stressor, particularly for children with severe medical conditions that are likely be exposed to potentially painful procedures on a daily basis.[6] Given the profound impact of pain on child and parent satisfaction and therefore compliance with healthcare delivery and services, and the documented unoptimal level of management, alternative and additional approaches to address the multidimensionality of pain represent a matter of urgency.

In the past decades, virtual-reality (VR) technology has been increasingly applied to healthcare in both the adult and pediatric context[7] where it has proven to be an accessible and helpful tool for a variety of purposes, including diagnosis and symptom management of several conditions,[8] medical education and training,[9] rehabilitation delivery,[10] and research. Three primary categories of VR simulations are currently available: nonimmersive, semi-immersive, and fully immersive.

Nonimmersive virtual experiences provide a monitor-generated environment (for example, from a computer or a console) where the user is allowed stay aware and in control of their real world. This VR is now commonly in use in everyday life.

Semi-immersive virtual experiences offer interaction with a partially virtual environment (for example, projectors or hard simulators), offering the user the perception of being in a different reality when focusing on the digital image while remaining connected to their physical surroundings.

Fully immersive simulations allow the user to experience a multisensorial virtual environment, with the user typically wearing glasses or a head-mounted display and interacting with the virtual world as if they were really in it. It represents the most realistic experience and the category on which we focus in this chapter. In pediatric inpatient and outpatient care, it is common to apply distraction techniques such as using toys or play in order to reduce the child's discomfort during medical procedures. The benefit seems to be greater for interactive distraction (e.g., playing a video game) opposed to passive (e.g., watching a video game) strategies.[11] The use of VR is particularly suitable to create a dynamic and personalized environment, contributing to ensuring a child-friendly healthcare approach.

In children, the most commonly, and first, explored use of VR has focused on pain management and pain-related distress, investigating VR as a distraction treatment to reduce acute pain, fear, anxiety, and stress during invasive medical procedures and chronic pain with protocols applying different technologies.[12]

Trost et al. described the VR approaches to pain and discussed the three interrelated dimensions of VR as presence, immersion, and interactivity.[13] Presence is the "subjective experience of being in one place or environment, even when one is physically situated in another."[14] This feeling together with the immersion refers to the user's sense of being engaged and captivated by the digital audiovisual content is related to exposure and distraction, which are the principal drivers of the user's changes in the cognitive, emotional, and social behaviors.

All these points together with the interactivity which is maybe the most important aspect of the VR experience, are involved in distraction which is one of the principal aspects evaluated in the use of immersive technology in pediatrics.

Despite some positive reports,[15] the effectiveness of VR in relieving acute and immediate pain remains uncertain.[16] However, studies on the long-term benefits of treating chronic pain are lacking, likely because this technology was particularly expensive until a few years ago. Distraction is one of the fundamental processes of VR, whereas an increased level of distraction coincides with a greater degree of involvement or agency.[17] Two other fundamental qualities underlying immersive virtual reality (VR) are the shifting of attention from the real world to the world occurring in the viewer (focus shifting) and the potential development of skills (skill building), a mechanism that assists patients in developing the necessary skills to regulate their response to painful stimuli and to be protagonists in their treatment path.[18]

Its application to palliative care (PC) has just recently started to receive attention,[19] with only a few efforts for children and adolescents with pediatric palliative-care (PPC) needs. VR can offer several potential advantages for pediatric patients with

Life-threatening conditions for which curative care may be feasible but can fail	Conditions which lead to premature deaths characterised by period of intensive treatments aimed to prolonging life
Progressive conditions without curative options with exclusive palliative treatment	Irreversible but nonprogressive conditions causing severe disability and likely premature death

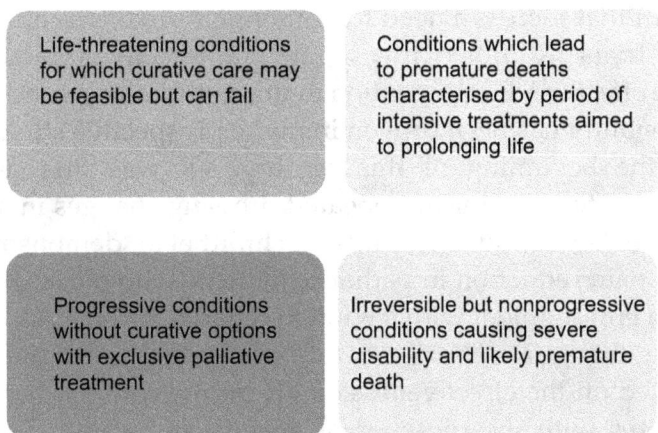

FIGURE 4.1 Four quadrant model developed by *Association for Children with Life-Threatening or Terminal Conditions and Their Families (ACT)* (now Together for Short Lives) to classify the conditions of children in pediatric palliative-care research.

oncological, genetic and metabolic disease, patients with neurologic life-limiting disease with disabilities and strong rehabilitation needs, as well improving their quality of life during and after treatment (see Figure 4.1).

Immersive Technology in Acute and Periprocedural Pain

Immersive technologies in acute and procedural pediatric pain have largely focused on preoperative and emergency department settings[20] to minimize children's pain and anxiety during invasive medical procedures such as burn wound care,[21] venipuncture,[22] lumbar puncture,[23] chemotherapy and port-access procedures in oncological patients,[24] and before surgery.[25] For some VR interventions, the content has been developed specifically for a certain procedure (e.g., *SnowWorld* and *Ice Cream Factory* in burn wound dressings).

Distraction through VR allows children experiencing pain to shift their attentional resources toward other stimuli with a hypoanalgesic effect[26] but most literature is focused on monocentric studies with small cohorts and many authors highlight that there is a need for larger high-quality randomized control trials (RCTs) to investigate the effectiveness and the adverse effect of VR intervention in this population), considering that feasibility has been proven in many prospective studies.

At the beginning of this century, VR was first used to manage acute pain during repeated dressing changes in adolescent patients with burn wounds.[27] Schmitt et al. demonstrated a 27–44% pain reduction in pediatric patients who participated in a virtual environment with a winter scenario, *SnowWorld*, during dressing changes.[28] Thanks to this result, further studies were conducted on the effectiveness of VR in care contexts involving procedures with the presence of anxiety and pain.[29] The relevant literature mainly deals with procedures that require acupuncture, i.e., procedures such as the simple sampling of venous blood up to the positioning of central venous catheters with peripheral insertion.[30] What these studies have in common is the advantage that VR brings not only to the patient, but also to the caregiver and healthcare personnel carrying out the procedure.

Due to research studies done on the management of procedural pain, it has been discovered that observing one's own body parts—like the hands—appear in a virtual environment (referred to as the "embodied world") and blocking out external sounds causes the patient to become less aware of unpleasant stimuli and, as a result, experience less pain.[31]

According to a recent and comprehensive review, data are difficult to pool due to high heterogeneity in interventions, comparison methods, participants, size of the study, settings, and outcome measures, consistency of findings, therefore it seems unclear to whether virtual-reality distraction makes a difference to pain intensity in children undergoing clinical treatments and procedures and difficult to interpret the benefits or lack of benefits of VR distraction for acute pain in children.[32] However, children who received a VR intervention were twice as satisfied with their pain management as compared to children not exposed to a VR intervention. Future well-designed, large, high-quality trials are needed to bring clarity on these conflicting findings.

A particular focus that has not yet been deeply investigated is the application of VR in pain management in procedures aimed at patients with chronic conditions as oncological patients. Given the repeated harm that can occur if pain is not adequately treated, it is important to consider once more in these children the use of alternative strategies for managing pain, beyond standard care. Some reports in the literature are focusing on potential benefits of VR technology during radiotherapy and intrathecal procedures as supportive treatment enhancing their quality of life. A close collaboration between researchers, clinicians, and VR experts is needed to identify and promote the right content and way to deliver VR technology in more clinical procedures.[33]

Immersive Technology in Chronic Pain Management

The role of immersive technologies in pediatric pain is not only to provide distraction from pain, but also uses biofeedback, graded exposure, and motivation that can be helpful in order to give more resources to patients who face chronic pain.[34] Many authors applied VR in patients with chronic pain stating that it is well tolerated and easy to use.[35] The INOVATE-Pain consortium has outlined guiding principles for VR interventions in pediatric chronic pain with suggested measures and study procedures focusing mainly on measurements of quality of life and pain reduction. However, more comparative studies are needed in order to assess the improvement related to biofeedback stimulation in comparison with other instruments and technology. Relaxation and stress relief are some of the benefits reported by patients using VR in chronic pain and these results also suggest a possible implementation in home-care setting using these techniques. Shiri et al. reported that combining VR with biofeedback to treat chronic headache in teenagers resulted in favorable benefits immediately, one month, and three months after intervention.[36] Griffin et al.,[37] for example, suggested an innovative VR program for juvenile pain therapy to promote improved upper and lower extremity involvement. The daily multisession reports revealed reduced pain, anxiety, avoidance, and functional deficits throughout VR sessions, which is consistent with previous research.[38] VR in pain rehabilitation assisted kids with chronic pain in a program in increasing pain distraction and improving function in order to fulfill rehabilitation goals.

After the COVID-19 pandemic, the possibilities related to telemedicine to offer telehealth sessions remotely should be explored in the near future trying to understand the role of immersive technology for managing pain using also remote VR by children at home.

Immersive Technology in Palliative Care

People suffering from terminal illnesses may have many and complicated physical and mental-health demands. VR may have an adjuvant nonpharmacological role in the therapy of complicated symptoms. VR in adult PC has been offered to end-of-life patients helping to control difficult symptoms such as pain, tiredness, drowsiness, shortness of breath, and depression, and enhancing psychological well-being and improving memory and legacy creation. To date, limited sample sizes and very low-quality studies, often without a comparator arm, have been reported. A recent review and meta-analysis conducted by Mo et al. reports eight studies analyzing the efficacy and feasibility of VR in adult inpatient palliative-care patients.[39] Moutogiannis et al. reviewed 14 articles describing VR use especially in advanced care patients where this approach creates an environment that allows the patients to be transported into a place they may not have been able to visit, or to be connected to families and childhood memories.[40]

These reviews suggest that recruitment was feasible and the intervention was enjoyable by patients with no adverse reactions noted but no study addressed the cost-effectiveness of VR compared to the efficacy and there were no standardized specific outcomes and measures used.[41] For palliative-care patients, different symptoms and conditions could potentially be positively affected by the exposure to immersive technology; somatic and psychological outcomes should be better defined and then analyzed in further studies. Pain (acute and chronic),[42] psychological well-being and mental-health problems (anxiety, depression and stress)[43] are poorly pointed out[44] whereas feasibility, acceptability, and usability, which are in general all reached, are more easily described. All immediate and indirect expenses related with VR, such as connectivity and staff training, are not reported as a crucial part of the program development.

PPC also deals with the physical, psychosocial, and spiritual concerns of patients and their families during end of life. This tool can be applied also in this context, in the perspective of taking care of children with other life-limiting conditions offering to clinicians a nonpharmacological resource to control the symptoms.[45]

Few reports are describing the use of VR for oncological pediatric patients during end of life.[46] A potentially interesting approach, which is not largely described in the adult population, is the possibility to provide immersive technology also in home care.[47]

The PPC setting poses unique challenges against the endless possibilities of VR usage.

The A.V.A.T.A.R. (Application of Virtual and Augmented realiTy in Palliative caRe) Project

PC in pediatrics is described as "the active overall care of the child's health, mind, and spirit, while also providing family support."[48]

PPC should be used as soon as an incurable or life-threatening condition is diagnosed, rather than only toward the end of life, and for this reason it differs from adult PC, due to the broad spectrum of diseases involved and the complexity of the consequent management for healthcare professionals and for the family members. At the moment, over 20 million children globally are eligible for PPC, and this figure is expected to rise over the next decade.[49] However, some key challenges remain when attempting to determine PPC demands. Our PPC referral center in Padua (Italy) serves more than 300 children and families facing life-limiting and life-threatening conditions in the Veneto area. Our service provide care both at the inpatient pediatric hospice, in the pediatric department and at home. Our multidisciplinary team, including pediatricians, physical and rehabilitation physiscian, physiotherapists, nurses, and psychologists, is also accessible 24/7 to oversee the care of PPC-eligible patients in regional community care hospitals. Our pain service also provides chronic pain consultations and non-operating room anesthesia (NORA) for pediatric patients of our department, counting around 2,500 to 3,000 sedations a year.

We define in our setting three possible applications areas of VR:

◆ *Acute and procedural pain*: Painful procedures are often necessary as part of diagnostic and treatment strategies for various medical conditions in children. In the past few years, a multimodal pain management approach has been developed, suggesting different pharmacological and nonpharmacological interventions; among them, immersive VR has emerged as one of the most promising tools for painful and stressful medical procedures.

◆ *Relief of anxiety and uncomfortable feelings related to chronic pain*: Some patients followed by our center also experience chronic pain or difficult neuroirritative symptoms such as dystonia, reporting pain on most days, had significantly greater functional disability and depressive symptoms. VR can provide a fully immersive experience, allowing patients to explore and interact with nature or other positive inputs in a 360-degree world right from their home in order to make these moments more tolerable and/or to have some relief during a pain crisis.

◆ *Benefits for psychological well-being of healthcare providers*: VR could play a role in alleviating the numerous stressors to which healthcare providers (HCPs) are exposed during long shifts and in limiting the related psychoemotional consequences.[50]

PPC providers experience considerable psychological distress while caring for children with life-threatening and life-limiting illnesses. They are responsible for ensuring the quality of life, alleviating suffering of the child and family, and guiding decision making in complex or critical situations involving end-of-life care and bereavement after the child's death.[51] These professionals are therefore continuously exposed to demanding emotional situations/phenomena that may increase their emotional burden and disrupt both the personal well-being and job performance.[52] Studies relating to the COVID-19 pandemic have widely confirmed that the healthcare sector is in itself characterized by the presence of psychosocial risk factors.[53] Especially during the recent pandemic, healthcare workers have had to cope with emotional overload and heavy workloads, shortage of adequate personal protective equipment, physical fatigue, and in some cases, organizational issues and changes in practices and procedures. Other emotional factors were related to high patient mortality, the suffering for loss of patients and colleagues, and an often prolonged separation from family.[54] The first studies in the literature regarding the use of VR for treatment of stress and burnout among healthcare professionals date back precisely to the post-COVID period. To verify the feasibility of immersive VR among PPC providers, we designed a single-arm pilot study involving our multidisciplinary team at the Veneto Regional Center for Pediatric Palliative Care (Italy) and obtained preliminary data about immersive VR efficacy and safety on the psychological distress of this population.[55] First, we investigated their baseline psychological profile and burden in the form of anxiety and moral distress through self-administered selected questionnaires. The immersive VR intervention was then provided through Oculus Quest 2, composed of a headset and two one-handed controllers (Facebook Technologies LLC) and consisted of a ten-minute session of a free demo version of the TRIPP mindfulness app at the end of daywork. This mindfulness app aims to induce relaxation by providing a fully immersive meditation experience (TRIPP Inc, Los Angeles, California, USA). Before starting the practice, the participants were asked through the app to self-rate their mood and emotions with a numerical (0 to 10) and a smiley face scale, respectively. Once the experience ended, we asked them to express some additional comments. Despite the singular-session design of our study, our results supported VR as a feasible and effective approach for improving mood and feelings, even in a high-burden population as the one working in PPC.

Limitations and Challenges of Virtual-Reality Application and Research

The problems and difficulties associated with the implementation of VR are frequently highlighted in the literature.[56] There have been five Cochrane reviews investigating the potential therapeutic benefits of VR: in pediatric pain,[57] rehabilitation following a stroke[58] and multiple sclerosis,[59] for people with Parkinson Disease[60] and serious mental illness.[61] All reported that it was difficult to make recommendations for clinical practice due to low-quality studies and low strength of evidence; all advocated for larger trials. First of all, methodological and clinical challenges need to be addressed in terms of more rigorous study designs, and standardized outcome measures are needed to improve the quality of the evidence. However, we also need more clinical definitions of outcomes. In the context of PC, for example, the exploration of acute pain versus chronic pain versus symptoms potentially describing disease progression is mandatory to define and understand the therapeutic efficacy of using VR.[62]

In most RCTs, researchers analyze physiological outcomes to define the benefit of a pain-related therapy together with psychological scale rating anxiety, burn out, and/or stress, but in many cases these aspects are not explored carefully and a parent's evaluation is also not so frequent. Giving voice to patient-oriented outcomes and how these changes are really impacting everyday life will lead to more measures and considerably more valuable outcomes.

Secondly, appropriate policy measures should be standardized and considered to guarantee that the platforms and experiences are monitored for content and quality, in order to avoid adverse effects such as nausea or dizziness. The creation of VR environments may be expensive and needs a team of specialists.[63] We may categorize these problems into technical problems and unique difficulties associated with the pediatric age, particularly in the setting of pediatric patients.

VR should be employed in clinical treatment, but there is currently no clear guidance on how to do so. We propose a checklist considering the steps to safely provide an adequate VR experience to children and young adults considering three different phases (pre-experience phase, VR experience, and postexperience phase, Table 4.1). One of the principal issues, and especially after the pandemic, is that the infection control and the institutional and organizational process necessary to ensure the VR to be used

Task	Who	
Adequate training for the staff	VR specialist—VR team physicians psychologists physiotherapists occupational therapist	Before the Experience
Define the outcomes and scales (pre-test)	Physicians Psychologists	
Check: the connectivity requirements the equipment is charged the headphones and visor can work independently	VR specialist—VR team	
Apply infection control regulation	VR specialist—VR team	
Choose the right device for the right child (size, form..) and the right software for the right experience	VR specialist—VR team	
Pre-briefing for the child and the parent: remote operation and second screen viewing (mirroring)	VR specialist—VR team	During the Experience
Assisting the patient during the experience	VR specialist—VR team	
Measure the outcomes (post test)	Physicians Psychologists	After the Experience

TABLE 4.1 Checklist for safe and easy use of VR in pediatrics

safely, effectively, and sustainably in many hospitals do not exist yet. This is also related to limited VR application, which is still in the clinical field, and to the fact that the number of devices is still limited in most of hospitals. This is connected to the few applications that are still being used in the clinical setting as well as the fact that there aren't many devices available in the majority of hospitals. We show the principle limitation to the use of VR in Figure 4.2.

A proper introduction to the technology prior to the experience is one of the most common technical problems mentioned by both adult and pediatric patients. Patients frequently mention in the evaluation form how difficult it was for them to operate certain parts of the VR device independently and how much help they needed. This is a key element in empowering the patient and enabling them to have an independent and autonomous experience, considering that in the pediatric patient, especially for children below the age of 12, parental assistance or a dedicated operator is mandatory. In order to monitor the experience, particularly in pediatrics, it can be helpful to guide the child in using the VR device and remote operation; second screen viewing

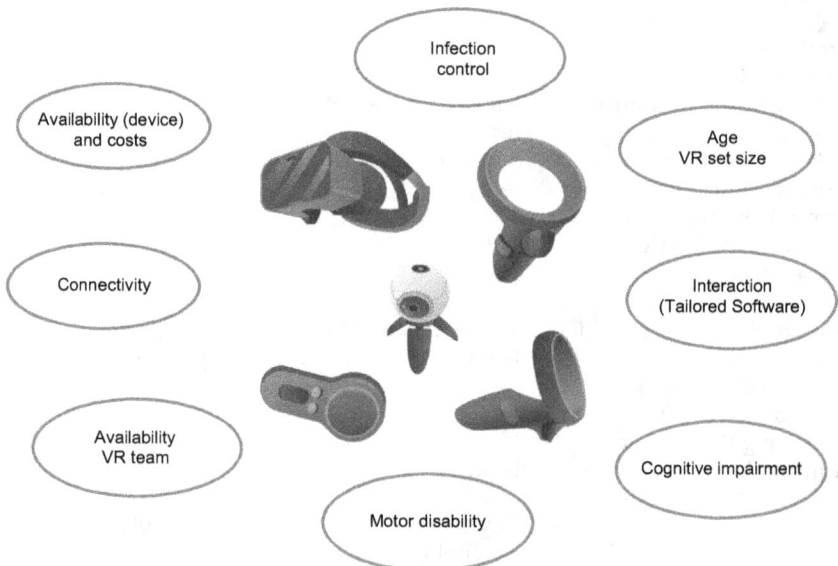

FIGURE 4.2 Limitation to VR use.

(mirroring) is also a useful resource, but the operator needs to remain with the participant throughout the entire experience.

Regardless of the application used, regular software upgrades are typically necessary; thus, it is essential to ensure the device is updated before usage. Verify that each gadget is being charged independently, including the headphones and visor if needed. Finally, the ability to access hospital intranet networking and access to the internet is tied to the health information technology department's organized support of ward applications and consideration of the use of VR in hospital PC. Numerous publications noted issues that precluded the adoption of VR,[64] and this may be even more crucial in the context of home care. Cellular mobile internet's ability to build hotspots has been exploited on these occasions, although it has had a negative impact on the video quality.

The availability of age-, patient-, and culturally appropriate VR applications, size and weight of the headsets, patient isolation status, and infection control consideration are factors to discuss further with industry partnerships and collaborations to leverage co-design and co-development. The headset size may cause headaches and eye aches, as most devices' interpupillary distance is designed for older children and adults. As such, most headset developers recommend only children over eight years old to use VR. However, there has been no evidence provided on the effects of VR on younger children. As a result, concerns regarding the use of VR in younger children still exist.

Future Directions

The future of VR is increasingly leaning toward multisensory experiences, and technology development is growing in this sense. The users can integrate visual stimulus with the possibility to touch, smell, and even taste. The more realistic the virtual world, the more immersive and captivating the experience for the user.

In healthcare, both patients and carers can enjoy the benefits of being in an immersive environment. To deepen that sense of immersion, the devices will become cheaper and lighter, removing the friction that can currently be a barrier and enlarging in this sense the potential number of users. VR for relaxation can be an intervention accessible to healthcare workers even during their work shift. The impact of long-term use will be an area of interest for further research.

Another interesting application of VR for healthcare professionals is as a training tool: It can provide a rich, interactive, and immersive training context that supports experiential learning through action.[65] The increased interest and motivation of trainees and the support in the acquisition and transfer of skills are crucial steps to empower healthcare in effective training. In this way, the learning process can be resolved within an experiential framework.

VR gamification is a fast-developing sector of technology that allows users to interact with virtual worlds and immersive game experiences. It entails incorporating computer-generated simulations, or virtual environments, into an interactive game.

Players in VR games may interact with their surroundings. This type of user engagement creates a one-of-a-kind and engaging experience that promotes exploration, problem-solving, and learning. Furthermore, players are awarded with points or other benefits for accomplishing objectives within the game. These incentives encourage people to keep playing and advance in the game.

VR gamification, in addition to offering an immersive experience, motivates players to fulfill certain objectives or activities in order to move farther in the game.[66] This increases incentive and keeps players interested and actively engaging in the game. Furthermore, these objectives may be adjusted so that each user gets a personalized experience that boosts the chance of them completing the activity at hand.[67]

Finally, VR gamification allows developers to track user behavior in real time and find areas for development. With this information, developers may make improvements to ensure that all players have a positive gaming experience, regardless of the state of development their game is in.

Existing game-based VR programs as well as rehabilitation-centered VR programs do not currently meet all the needs of pediatric patients in regard to defining pain and or other specific somatic outcomes. To address this opportunity for meaningful VR engagement in rehabilitation, there is a need to implement software and have specific designed applications as shown by Griffin et al.[68]

VR games may be employed as an effective and captivating treatment by engaging the child with artificial scenes, objects, and events that seem and feel like real-world scenarios. It has been shown to improve focus and motivation for therapeutic goals.[69] According to some randomized studies, individuals who got gamified-VR rehabilitation therapy had better pain reduction, especially those who had severe pain at the start has been proved.[70]

References

1 Shomaker, K., Dutton, S., & Mark, M. (2015). Pain prevalence and treatment patterns in a US children's hospital. *Hospital Pediatrics*, *5*(7), 363–370; Stevens, B.J., Harrison, D., Rashotte, J., Yamada, J., Abbott, L.K., Coburn, G., Stinson, J., & Le May, S. (2012). Pain assessment and intensity in hospitalized children in Canada. *Journal of Pain*, *13*(9), 857–865; Walther-Larsen, S., Pedersen, M.T., Friis, S.M., Aagaard, G.B., Romsing, J., Jeppesen, E.M., & Friedrichsdorf, S.J. (2016). Pain prevalence in hospitalized children: A prospective cross-sectional survey in four Danish university hospitals. *Acta Anaesthesiologica Scandinavica*.

2 Birnie, K.A., Chambers, C.T., Fernandez, C.V., Forgeron, P.A., Latimer, M.A., McGrath, P.J., Cummings, E.A., & Finley, G.A. (2014). Hospitalized children continue to report undertreated and preventable pain. *Pain Research & Management, 19*(4), 198–204; Friedrichsdorf, S.J., Postier, A., Eull, D., Weidner, C., Foster, L., Gilbert, M., & Campbell, F. (2015). Pain outcomes in a US children's hospital: A prospective cross-sectional survey. *Hospital Pediatrics, 5*(1), 18–26; Twycross, A., & Collis, S. (2013). How well is acute pain in children managed?

A snapshot in one English hospital. *Pain Management Nursing, 14*(4), e204–215; Friedrichsdorf, S.J., & Goubert, L. (2019, December 19) Pediatric pain treatment and prevention for hospitalized children. *Pain Reports, 5*(1), e80.

3 Williams, A.C., & Craig, K.D. (2016). Updating the definition of pain. *Pain, 157,* 2420–2423; International Association for the Study of Pain (IASP). (n.d.). Pain terms: A current list with definitions and notes on usage: Recommended by the IASP subcommittee on taxonomy. Retrieved from https://www.iasp-pain.org/terminology? navItemNumber=576 2011

4 Aydede, M. (2017). Defending the IASP definition of pain. *Monist, 100*(4), 439–464.

5 McGrath, P.J., Walco, G.A., Turk, D.C., Dworkin, R.H., Brown, M.T., Davidson, K., et al. (2008). Core outcome domains and measures for pediatric acute and chronic/recurrent pain clinical trials: PedIMMPACT recommendations. *Journal of Pain, 9*(9), 771–783; Blount, R.L., Piira, T., Cohen, L.L., & Cheng, P.S. (2006). Pediatric procedural pain. *Behavior Modification, 30*(1), 24–49.

6 Fox, J.K., Halpern, L.F., Dangman, B.C., Giramonti, K.M., & Kogan, B.A. (2016). Children's anxious reactions to an invasive medical procedure: The role of medical and non-medical fears. *Journal of Health Psychology, 21*(8), 1587–1596; Quinn, B.L., Solodiuk, J.C., Morrill, D., & Mauskar, S. (2018, August 11). Pain in nonverbal children with medical complexity: A two-year retrospective study. *American Journal of Nursing, 118*(8), 28–37.

7 Chirico, A., Lucidi, F., De Laurentiis, M., et al. (2016). Virtual reality in health system: Beyond entertainment. A mini-review on the efficacy of VR during cancer treatment. *Journal of Cellular Physiology, 231,* 275–287; Yeung, A.W.K., Tosevska, A., Klager, E., Eibensteiner, F., Laxar, D., Stoyanov, J., Glisic, M., Zeiner, S., Kulnik, S.T., Crutzen, R., Kimberger, O., Kletecka-Pulker, M., Atanasov, A.G., & Willschke, H. (2021, February 10). Virtual and augmented reality applications in medicine: Analysis of the scientific literature. *Journal of Medical Internet Research, 23*(2), e25499; Cheng, Z., Yu, S., Zhang, W., Liu, X., Shen, Y., & Weng, H. (2022, September 28). Virtual reality for pain and anxiety of pediatric oncology patients: A systematic review and meta-analysis. *Asia-Pacific Journal of Oncology Nursing, 9*(12), 100152; Addab, S., Hamdy, R., Thorstad, K., Le May, S., & Tsimicalis, A.

(2022, November). Use of virtual reality in managing paediatric procedural pain and anxiety: An integrative literature review. *Journal of Clinical Nursing, 31*(21–22), 3032–3059, epub 2022, January 23; Hoag, J.A., Karst, J., Bingen, K., Palou-Torres, A., & Yan, K. (2022, April 18). Distracting through procedural pain and distress using virtual reality and guided imagery in pediatric, adolescent, and young adult patients: Randomized controlled trial. *Journal of Medical Internet Research, 24*(4), e30260.

8 Oyama, H. (1997). Virtual reality for the palliative care of cancer. *Studies in Health Technology and Informatics, 144*, 87–94; Schneider, S.M., & Hood, L.E. (2007). Virtual reality: A distraction intervention for chemotherapy. *Oncology Nursing Forum, 34*, 39–46.

9 Yeung, A.W.K., Tosevska, A., Klager, E., Eibensteiner, F., Laxar,D., Stoyanov, J., Glisic, M., Zeiner, S., Kulnik, S.T., Crutze,n R., Kimberger, O., Kletecka-Pulker, M., Atanasov, A.G., & Willschke, H. (2021, February 10). Virtual and augmented reality applications in medicine: Analysis of the scientific literature. *Journal of Medical Internet Research, 23*(2), e25499; Mergen, M., Meyerheim, M., & Graf, N. (2023, June 20). Reviewing the current state of virtual reality integration in medical education: A scoping review protocol. *Systematic Review, 12*(1), 97.

10 Laver, K.E., Lange, B., George, S., Deutsch, J.E., Saposnik, G., & Crotty, M. (2017). Virtual reality for stroke rehabilitation. *Cochrane Database of Systematic Reviews, 11*. Art. no. CD008349. https:// doi.org/10.1002/14651858.CD008349.pub4; De Keersmaecker, E., Beckwée, D., Denissen, S., Nagels, G., & Swinnen, E. (2020). Virtual reality for multiple sclerosis rehabilitation (Protocol). *Cochrane Database of Systematic Reviews, 12*. Art. no.: CD013834. https://doi .org/10.1002/14651858.CD013834

11 De Keersmaecker, E., Beckwée, D., Denissen, S., Nagels, G., & Swinnen, E. (2020). Virtual reality for multiple sclerosis rehabilitation (Protocol). *Cochrane Database of Systematic Reviews, 12*. Art. no.: CD013834. https://doi.org/10.1002/14651858.CD013834

12 Wohlheiter, K.A., & Dahlquist, L.M. (2013). Interactive versus passive distraction for acute pain management in young children: The role of selective attention and development. *Journal of Pediatric Psychology, 38*(2), 202–212.

13 Trost, Z., France, C., Anam, M., & Shum, C. (2021). Virtual reality approaches to pain: Toward a state of the science. *Pain, 162*(2), 325–331.

14 Trost, Z., France, C., Anam, M., & Shum, C. (2021). Virtual reality approaches to pain: Toward a state of the science. *Pain, 162*(?), 325–331.

15 Merino-Lobato, C., Rodríguez-Gallego, I., Pabón-Carrasco, M., Romero-Castillo, R., & Jiménez-Picón, N. (2023, November–December). Virtual reality vs. buzzy® efficacy in pain and anxiety management during pediatric venipuncture. Systematic review and meta-analysis. *Journal of Pediatric Nursing, 73*, 22–33. https://doi.org/10.1016/j.pedn.2023.08.014; Tas, F.Q., van Eijk, C.A.M., Staals, L.M., Legerstee, J.S., & Dierckx, B. (2022, December). Virtual reality in pediatrics, effects on pain and anxiety: A systematic review and meta-analysis update. *Paediatric Anaesthesia, 32*(12), 1292–1304. https://doi.org/10.1111/pan.14546

16 Kenney, M.P., & Milling, L.S. (2016). The effectiveness of virtual reality distraction for reducing pain: A meta-analysis. *Psychology of Consciousness: Theory, Research and Practice, 3*(3), 199–210.

17 Pourmand, A., Davis, S., Marchak, A., Whiteside, T., & Sikka, N. (2018, June 15). Virtual reality as a clinical tool for pain management. *Current Pain and Headache Reports, 22*(8), 53.

18 Garrett, B., Taverner, T., Masinde, W., Gromala, D., Shaw, C., & Negraeff, M. (2014, December). A Rapid evidence assessment of immersive virtual reality as an adjunct therapy in acute pain management in clinical practice. *Clinical Journal of Pain, 30*(12), 1089–1098.

19 Martin, J.L., Saredakis, D., Hutchinson, A.D., Crawford, G.B., & Loetscher, T. (2022, June 29). Virtual reality in palliative Care: A systematic review. *Healthcare* (Basel), *10*(7), 1222; Brennan, P.F., Arnott Smith, C., Ponto, K., Radwin, R., & Kreutz, K. (2013). Envisioning the future of home care: Applications of immersive virtual reality. *Studies in Health Technology and Informatics, 192*, 599–602.

20 Lambert, V., Boylan, P., Boran, L., Hicks, P., Kirubakaran, R., Devane, D., et al. (2020). Virtual reality distraction for acute pain in children. *Cochrane Database of Systematic Reviews, 10*, 11–13.

21 Hoffman, H.G., Patterson, D.R., Seibel, E., Soltani, M., Jewett-Leahy, L., & Sharar, S.R. (2008). Virtual reality pain control during burn wound debridement in the hydrotank. *Clinical Journal of Pain, 24*(4), 299–304.

22 Wong, C.L, & Choi, K.C. (2023, February 1). Effects of an immersive virtual reality intervention on pain and anxiety among pediatric patients undergoing venipuncture: A randomized clinical

trial. *JAMA Network Open, 6*(2), e230001. https://doi.org/10.1001/ jamanetworkopen.2023.0001

23 Wint, S.S., Eshelman, D., Steele, J., & Guzzetta, C.E. (2002). Effects of distraction using virtual reality glasses during lumbar punctures in adolescents with cancer. *Oncology Nursing Forum, 9*(1), e8–15.

24 Oyama, H. (1997). Virtual reality for the palliative care of cancer. *Studies in Health Technology and Informatics, 144,* 87–94; Schneider, S.M., & Hood, L.E. (2007). Virtual reality: A distraction intervention for chemotherapy. *Oncology Nursing Forum, 34,* 39–46; Ahmadi, M. (2001). Virtual reality may help children under-going chemotherapy. *Journal of the National Cancer Institute, 93,* 675–676; Rygh, L., Johal, S., Johnson, H., & Karlson, C.W. (2023, November–December). Virtual Reality for pediatric oncology port-a-cath access: A pilot effectiveness study. *Journal of Pediatric Hematology/Oncology Nursing, 40*(6), 379–385. https://doi .org/10.1177/27527530221147875

25 Esposito, C., Autorino, G., Iervolino, A., Vozzella, E.A., Cerulo, M., Esposito, G., Coppola, V., Carulli, R., Cortese, G., Gallo, L., & Escolino, M. (2022, February). Efficacy of a virtual reality program in pedi-atric surgery to reduce anxiety and distress symptoms in the pre-operative phase: A Prospective randomized clinical trial. *Journal of Laparoendoscopic & Advanced Surgical Techniques, Part A, 32*(2), 197–203. https://doi.org/10.1089/lap.2021.0566; Ryu, J.H., Park, J.W., Nahm, F.S., Jeon, Y.T., Oh, A.Y., Lee, H.J., Kim, J.H., & Han, S.H. (2018, September). The effect of gamification through a virtual reality on preoperative anxiety in pediatric patients undergoing general anesthesia: A prospective, randomized, and controlled trial. *Journal of Clinical Medicine, 7*(9), 284. https://doi.org/10.3390/jcm7090284

26 Persky, S., & Lewis, M.A. (2019, November 25). Advancing science and practice using immersive virtual reality: What behavioral medi-cine has to offer. *Translational Behavioral Medicine, 9*(6), 1040–1046.

27 Hoffman, H.G., Patterson, D.R., Seibel, E., Soltani, M., Jewett-Leahy, L., & Sharar, S.R. (2008). Virtual reality pain control during burn wound debridement in the hydrotank. *Clinical Journal of Pain, 24*(4), 299–304; Hoffman, H.G., Doctor, J.N., Patterson, D.R., Carrougher, G.J., & Furness, T.A.I. (2000, March 1). Virtual reality as an adjunctive pain control during burn wound care in adolescent patients. *Pain, 85*(1), 305–309.

28 Schmitt, Y.S., Hoffman, H.G., Blough, D.K., Patterson, D.R, Jensen, M.P., Soltani, M., et al. (2011, February). A randomized, controlled trial of immersive virtual reality analgesia, during physical therapy for pediatric burns. *Burns: Journal of the International Society for Burn Injuries, 37*(1), 61–68.

29 Persky, S., & Lewis, M.A. (2019, November 25). Advancing science and practice using immersive virtual reality: What behavioral medicine has to offer. *Translational Behavioral Medicine, 9*(6), 1040–1046.

30 Won, A.S., Bailey, J., Bailenson, J., Tataru, C., Yoon, I.A., & Golianu, B. (2017, July). Immersive virtual reality for pediatric pain. *Children, 4*(7), 52.

31 Won, A.S., Bailey, J., Bailenson, J., Tataru, C., Yoon, I.A., & Golianu, B. (2017, July). Immersive virtual reality for pediatric pain. *Children, 4*(7), 52.

32 Lambert, V., Boylan, P., Boran, L., Hicks, P., Kirubakaran, R., Devane, D., et al. (2020). Virtual reality distraction for acute pain in children. *Cochrane Database of Systematic Reviews, 10.*

33 Yap, K.Y., Koh, D.W.H., Lee, V.S.J., & Wong, L.L. (2020, December). Use of virtual reality in the supportive care management of pediatric patients with cancer. *Lancet Child & Adolescent Health, 4*(12), 899–908. https://doi.org/10.1016/S2352–4642(20)30240-6; Alanazi, A., Ashour, F., Aldosari, H., & Aldosari, B. (2022, January 14). The impact of virtual reality in enhancing the quality of life of pediatric oncology patients. *Studies in Health Technology and Informatics, 289,* 477–480. https://doi.org/10.3233/SHTI210961

34 Griffin, A., Wilson, L., Feinstein, A.B., Bortz, A., Heirich, M.S., Gilkerson, R., et al. (2020). Virtual reality in pain rehabilitation for youth with chronic pain: Pilot feasibility study. *JMIR Rehabilitation and Assistive Technologies, 7*(2), e22620; Logan, D.E., Simons, L.E., Caruso, T., Gold, J.I., Griffin, A., King, C., et al. (2020). Leveraging VR/AR to combat chronic pain in youth: Position paper from the Interdisciplinary Network on Virtual and Augmented (AR/VR) Technologies for pain (INOVATE-Pain) management. *Journal of Medical Internet Research.*

35 Griffin, A., Wilson, L., Feinstein, A.B., Bortz, A., Heirich, M.S., Gilkerson, R., et al. (2020). Virtual reality in pain rehabilitation for youth with chronic pain: Pilot feasibility study. *JMIR Rehabilitation and Assistive Technologies, 7*(2), e22620.

36 Shiri, S., Feintuch, U., Weiss, N., Pustilnik, A., Geffen, T., Kay, B., Meiner, Z., & Berger, I. (2013, May). A virtual reality system combined

with biofeedback for treating pediatric chronic headache—A pilot study. *Pain Medicine*, *14*(5), 621–627.

37 Griffin, A., Wilson, L., Feinstein, A.B., Bortz, A., Heirich, M.S., Gilkerson, R., et al. (2020). Virtual reality in pain rehabilitation for youth with chronic pain: Pilot feasibility study. *JMIR Rehabilitation and Assistive Technologies*, *7*(2), e22620.

38 Shiri, S., Feintuch, U., Weiss, N., Pustilnik, A., Geffen, T., Kay, B., Meiner, Z., & Berger, I. (2013, May). A virtual reality system combined with biofeedback for treating pediatric chronic headache--a pilot study. *Pain Medicine*, *14*(5), 621–627; Agrawal, A.K., Robertson, S., Litwin, L., Tringale, E., Treadwell, M., Hoppe, C., et al. (2019, Feburary). Virtual reality as complementary pain therapy in hospitalized patients with sickle cell disease. *Pediatric Blood Cancer*, *66*(2), e27525.

39 Mo, J., Vickerstaff, V., Minton, O., Tavabie, S., Taubert, M., Stone, P., & White, N. (2022, July). How effective is virtual reality technology in palliative care? A systematic review and meta-analysis. *Palliative Medicine*, *36*(7), 1047–1058. https://doi.org/10.1177/02692163221099584

40 Moutogiannis, P.P., Thrift, J., Pope, J.K., Browning, M.H.E.M., McAnirlin, O., & Fasolino, T. (2023, December 1). A rapid review of the role of virtual reality in care delivery of palliative care and hospice. *Journal of Hospice Palliative Nursing*, *25*(6), 300–308. https://doi.org/10.1097/NJH.0000000000000983

41 Moutogiannis, P.P., Thrift, J., Pope, J.K., Browning, M.H.E.M., McAnirlin, O., & Fasolino, T. (2023, December). A rapid review of the role of virtual reality in care delivery of palliative care and hospice. *Journal of Hospice Palliative Nursing*, *25*(6), 300–308. https://doi.org/10.1097/NJH.0000000000000983

42 Guenther, M., Görlich, D., Bernhardt, F., et al. (2022). Virtual reality reduces pain in palliative care–A feasibility trial. *BMC Palliative Care, 21*, 169. Retrieved from https://doi.org/10.1186/s12904-022-01058-4; Burridge, N., Sillence, A., Teape, L., Clark, B., Bruce, E., Armoogum, J., Leloch, D., Spathis, A., & Etkind, S. (2023, September). Virtual reality reduces anxiety and pain in acute hospital palliative care: Service evaluation. *BMJ Supportive Palliative Care*. https://doi.org/10.1136/spcare-2023–004572

43 Weingarten, K., Macapagal, F., & Parker, D. (2020, January). Virtual reality: Endless potential in pediatric palliative care: A case report. *Journal of Palliative Medicine*, *23*(1), 147–149. https://doi.org/10.1089/jpm.2019.0207

44 Mo, J., Vickerstaff, V., Minton, O., Tavabie, S., Taubert, M., Stone, P., & White, N. (2022, July). How effective is virtual reality technoloqy in palliative care? A systematic review and meta-analysis. *Palliative Medicine, 36*(7), 1047–1058. https://doi.org/10.1177/02692163221099584

45 Mo, J., Vickerstaff, V., Minton, O., Tavabie, S., Taubert, M., Stone, P., & White, N. (2022, July). How effective is virtual reality technoloqy in palliative care? A systematic review and meta-analysis. *Palliative Medicine, 36*(7), 1047–1058. https://doi.org/10.1177/02692163221099584

46 Moutogiannis, P.P., Thrift, J., Pope, J.K., Browning, M.H.E.M., McAnirlin, O., & Fasolino, T. (2023, December). A rapid review of the role of virtual reality in care delivery of palliative care and hospice. *Journal of Hospice Palliative Nursing, 25*(6), 300–308. https://doi.org/10.1097/NJH.0000000000000983

47 Moscato, S., Sichi, V., Giannelli, A., Palumbo, P., Ostan, R., Varani, S., Pannuti, R., & Chiari, L. (2021, September 24). Virtual reality in home palliative care: Brief report on the effect on cancer-related symptomatology. *Frontiers in Psychology, 12*, 709154. https://doi.org/10.3389/fpsyg.2021.709154

48 Benini, F., Cauzzo, C., Congedi, S., Da Dalt, L., Cogo, P., Biscaglia, L., et al. (2019). Training in pediatric palliative care in Italy: Still much to do. *Annali dell'Istituto Superiore di Sanità, 55*, 240–245. Retrieved from https://doi.org/10.4415/ANN_19_03_07; Kavalieratos, D., Corbelli, J., Zhang, D., Dionne-Odom, J.N., Ernecoff, N.C., Hanmer, J., et al. (2016). Association between palliative care and patient and caregiver outcomes: A systematic review and meta-analysis. *JAMA, 316*, 2104–2114. Retrieved from https://doi.org/10.1001/jama.2016.16840; World Health Organization. (2023, June 1). Palliative care for children. *World Health Organization.* Retrieved from https://www.who.int/europe/news-room/fact-sheets/item/palliative-care-for-children

49 Benini, F., Bellentani, M., Reali, L., Lazzarin, P., De Zen, L., Pellegatta, F., Aprile, P.L., & Scaccabarozzi, G. (2021, January 7). An estimation of the number of children requiring pediatric palliative care in Italy. *Italian Journal of Pediatrics, 47*(1), 4. https://doi.org/10.1186/s13052-020-00952-y

50 Mercante, A., Zanin, A., Vecchi, L., De Tommasi, V., & Benini, F. (2024, January 7). Virtual reality intervention as support to paediatric

palliative care providers: A pilot study. *Acta Paediatric.* https://doi.org/10.1111/apa.17099

51 Rico-Mena, P., Güeita-Rodríguez, J., Martino-Alba, R., Castel-Sánchez, M., & Palacios-Ceña, D. (2023, April 9). The emotional experience of caring for children in pediatric palliative care: A qualitative study among a home-based interdisciplinary care team. *Children (Basel), 10*(4), 700. https://doi.org/10.3390/children10040700; Kase, S.M., Waldman, E.D., & Weintraub, A.S. (2019, June). A cross-sectional pilot study of compassion fatigue, burnout, and compassion satisfaction in pediatric palliative care providers in the United States. *Palliative Support Care, 17*(3), 269–275. https://doi.org/10.1017/S1478951517001237

52 Rourke, M.T. (2007). Compassion fatigue in pediatric palliative care providers. *Pediatric Clinics of North America, 54,* 631–644.

53 Croghan, I.T., Hurt, R.T., Fokken, S.C., Fischer, K.M., Lindeen, S.A., Schroeder, D.R., Ganesh, R., Ghosh, K., Bausek, N., & Bauer, B.A. (2023, April). Stress resilience program for health care professionals during a pandemic: A pilot program. *Workplace Health & Safety, 71*(4), 173–180. https://doi.org/10.1177/21650799221093775; Zhou, Q., Wang, J., Duan, W., & Ye, B. (2024, January 5). Editorial: Assessing and evaluating the psychosocial impact of the COVID-19 pandemic on anxiety and stress: Perspectives from East Asia. *Frontiers in Psychiatry, 14,* 1353718. https://doi.org/10.3389/fpsyt.2023.1353718

54 Kottler, J., Gingell, M.J., Khosla, S., Kordzikowski, M., Raszewski, R., Chestek, D., & Maki, K. (2023, July 21). Exploring physical and biological manifestations of burnout and posttraumatic stress disorder symptoms in healthcare workers: A scoping review protocol. *BMJ Open, 13*(7), e074887. https://doi.org/10.1136/bmjopen-2023-074887

55 Mercante, A., Zanin, A., Vecchi, L., De Tommasi, V., & Benini, F. (2024, January 7). Virtual reality intervention as support to paediatric palliative care providers: A pilot study. *Acta Paediatric.* https://doi.org/10.1111/apa.17099

56 Mo, J., Vickerstaff, V., Minton, O., Tavabie, S., Taubert, M., Stone, P., & White, N. (2022, July). How effective is virtual reality technology in palliative care? A systematic review and meta-analysis. *Palliative Medicine, 36*(7), 1047–1058. https://doi.org/10.1177/02692163221099584;

Moutogiannis, P.P., Thrift, J., Pope, J.K., Browning, M.H.E.M., McAnirlin, O., & Fasolino, T. (2023, December) A rapid review of the role of virtual reality in care delivery of palliative care and hospice. *Journal of Hospice Palliative Nursing, 25*(6), 300–308. https://doi.org/10.1097/NJH.0000000000000983

57 Lambert, V., Boylan, P., Boran, L., Hicks, P., Kirubakaran, R., Devane, D., et al. (2020). Virtual reality distraction for acute pain in children. *Cochrane Database of Systematic Reviews, 10.*

58 Laver, K.E., Lange, B., George, S., Deutsch, J.E., Saposnik, G., & Crotty, M. (2017). Virtual reality for stroke rehabilitation. *Cochrane Database of Systematic Reviews, 11.* Art. no. CD008349. https://doi.org/10.1002/14651858.CD008349.pub4

59 De Keersmaecker, E., Beckwée, D., Denissen, S., Nagels, G., & Swinnen, E. (2020). Virtual reality for multiple sclerosis rehabilitation (Protocol). *Cochrane Database of Systematic Reviews, 12.* Art. no.: CD013834. https://doi.org/10.1002/14651858.CD013834

60 Dockx, K., Bekkers, E.M.J., Van den Bergh, V., Ginis, P., Rochester, L., Hausdorff, J.M., Mirelman, A., & Nieuwboer, A. (2015). Virtual reality for rehabilitation in Parkinson's disease. *Cochrane Database of Systematic Reviews, 12.* Art. no.: CD010760. https://doi.org/10.1002/14651858.CD010760.pub2

61 Välimäki, M., Hätönen, H.M., Lahti, M.E., Kurki, M., Hottinen, A., Metsäranta, K., Riihimäki, T., & Adams, C.E. (2014). Virtual reality for treatment compliance for people with serious mental illness. *Cochrane Database of Systematic Reviews, 10.* Art. no.: CD009928. https://doi.org/10.1002/14651858.CD009928.pub2

62 Woo, O.K.L. (2023, October 2). Integrating knowledge, skills, and attitudes: Professional training required for virtual reality therapists in palliative care. *Frontiers in Medical Technology, 5,* 1268662. https://doi.org/10.3389/fmedt.2023.1268662

63 Woo, O.K.L. (2023, October 2). Integrating knowledge, skills, and attitudes: Professional training required for virtual reality therapists in palliative care. *Frontiers in Medical Technology, 5,* 1268662. https://doi.org/10.3389/fmedt.2023.1268662

64 Mo, J., Vickerstaff, V., Minton, O., Tavabie, S., Taubert, M., Stone, P., & White, N. (2022, July). How effective is virtual reality technology in palliative care? A systematic review and meta-analysis. *Palliative Medicine, 36*(7), 1047–1058. https://doi.org/10.1177/02692163221099584;

Moutogiannis, P.P., Thrift, J., Pope, J.K., Browning, M.H.E.M., McAnirlin, O., & Fasolino, T. (2023, December). A rapid review of the role of virtual reality in care delivery of palliative care and hospice. *Journal of Hospice Palliative Nursing, 25*(6), 300–308. https://doi.org/10.1097/NJH.0000000000000983

65 Schneider, S.M., & Hood, L.E. (2007). Virtual reality: A distraction intervention for chemotherapy. *Oncology Nursing Forum, 34*, 39–46; Yeung, A.W.K., Tosevska, A., Klager, E., Eibensteiner, F., Laxar,D., Stoyanov, J., Glisic, M., Zeiner, S., Kulnik, S.T., Crutze,n R., Kimberger, O., Kletecka-Pulker, M., Atanasov, A.G., & Willschke, H. (2021, February 10). Virtual and augmented reality applications in medicine: Analysis of the scientific literature. *Journal of Medical Internet Research, 23*(2), e25499.

66 Janssen, J., Verschuren, O., Renger, W.J., Ermers, J., Ketelaar, M., & Van Ee, R. (2017). Gamification in physical therapy: More than using games. *Pediatric Physical Therapy, 29*, 95–99.

67 Pimentel-Ponce, M., Romero-Galisteo, R.P., Palomo-Carrión, R., Pinero-Pinto, E., Merchán-Baeza, J.A., Ruiz-Muñoz, M., Oliver-Pece, J., & González-Sánchez, M. (2021, April 15). Gamification and neurological motor rehabilitation in children and adolescents: A systematic review. *Neurologia*, S0213–4853(21)00049-9. https://doi.org/10.1016/j.nrl.2021.02.011

68 Griffin, A., Wilson, L., Feinstein, A.B., Bortz, A., Heirich, M.S., Gilkerson, R., et al. (2020). Virtual reality in pain rehabilitation for youth with chronic pain: Pilot feasibility study. *JMIR Rehabilitation and Assistive Technologies, 7*(2), e22620.

69 Janssen, J., Verschuren, O., Renger, W.J., Ermers, J., Ketelaar, M., & Van Ee, R. (2017). Gamification in physical therapy: More than using games. *Pediatric Physical Therapy, 29*, 95–99.

70 Pimentel-Ponce, M., Romero-Galisteo, R.P., Palomo-Carrión, R., Pinero-Pinto, E., Merchán-Baeza, J.A., Ruiz-Muñoz, M., Oliver-Pece, J., & González-Sánchez, M. (2021, April 15). Gamification and neurological motor rehabilitation in children and adolescents: A systematic review. *Neurologia*, S0213–4853(21)00049-9. https://doi.org/10.1016/j.nrl.2021.02.011

5

Healing the Palliative Practitioner

Jose Ferrer Costa

Caring for those nearing the end of their lives is an emotionally taxing endeavor, and stress and burnout are common pitfalls for palliative-care workers. The question arises: Could emerging technologies like virtual reality (VR) offer a way to equip these dedicated professionals with the mental-health skills they need to persevere? In this chapter, I delve into this question based on my own experience leading a research project that explores the potential of VR training in alleviating work-related stress among palliative-care workers.

In collaboration with Nuria Morán Bueno, a fellow family and community medicine specialist with expertise in neurolinguistic programming and mindfulness, we embarked on a study focused on the use of VR to train palliative-care workers in skills like mindfulness, self-compassion, and emotional regulation. The goal was to explore whether such a technological approach could effectively mitigate job-related burnout and enhance the emotional resilience of these healthcare professionals.

The postintervention data was encouraging. There were statistically significant reductions in emotional exhaustion and depersonalization among participants, along with notable improvements in personal accomplishment, vigor, dedication, and absorption. Importantly, those who initially reported higher

DOI: 10.4324/9781032649771-5

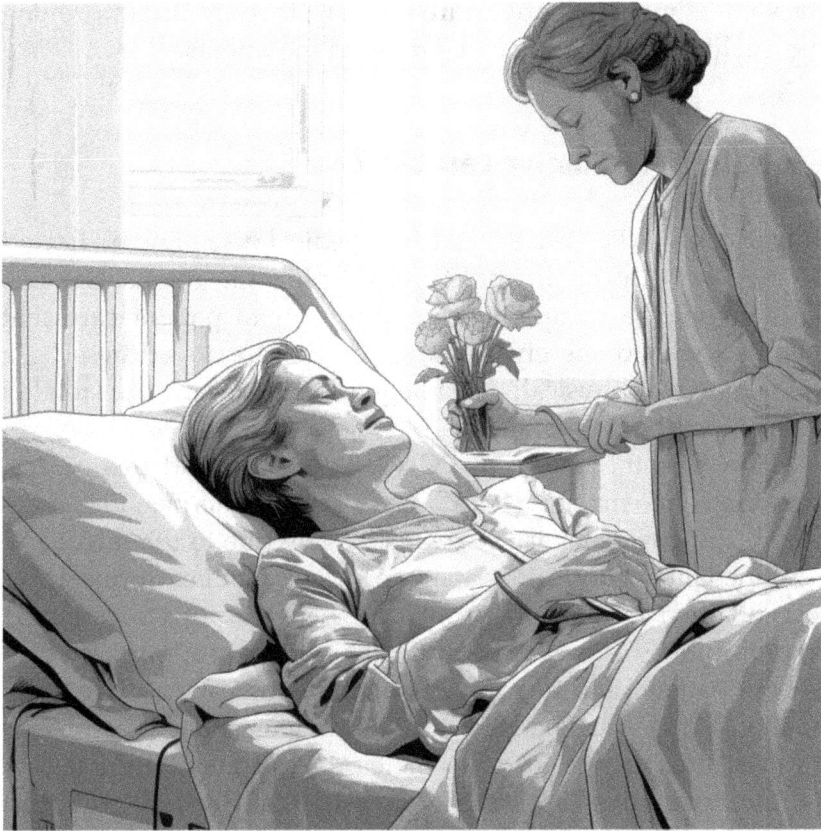

FIGURE 5.1

levels of work-related stress seemed to benefit the most from the program. The short virtual-reality program had a positive impact on the workers' burnout levels. They felt less emotionally exhausted and more accomplished after the training. They said that they felt more prepared to deal with the challenges that came their way and that they were more positive and engaged when working with their patients.

Our journey in developing this VR program has not only demonstrated its potential effectiveness but also showcased it as a cost-effective and accessible means of mental-health support. The results hint at a promising avenue for enhancing the well-being of palliative-care workers, thereby also improving the quality of end-of-life care provided to patients.

The Nature of Palliative-Care Work

Palliative care (PC) is a specialized medical discipline dedicated to improving the quality of life for people with serious illnesses. This involves a comprehensive approach to patient care that extends beyond merely treating the disease to addressing a broad range of physical, psychological, and social issues related to the illness.[1]

However, the nature of PC work goes beyond this clinical definition and encompasses a broad range of interpersonal, emotional, and psychological elements, largely due to the direct and sustained interaction with patients and their families during a critical and often terminal phase of illness. A significant aspect of their responsibilities centers on providing emotional support and care to both patients and their loved ones. The intensity and depth of relationships formed between health providers, patients, and their families often extend beyond a mere professional interaction.[2]

The palliative-care team comprises a diverse group of professionals including doctors, nurses, social workers, psychologists, occupational therapists, and spiritual advisors. This team collaborates closely to provide comprehensive patient care, offering symptom relief, emotional support, and help navigating the healthcare system. This interprofessional collaboration is key to the successful functioning of PC and adds a significant layer of complexity to the nature of PC work.

The importance of spirituality and religion is another unique facet of palliative-care work. For many patients and families, as well as for many members of the palliative-care team, spiritual beliefs offer a way to find meaning and comfort in the face of severe illness and death. This provides an additional dimension to palliative-care work, making it not only a clinical practice but also a deeply human interaction.[3]

Challenges in Making End-of-Life Decisions

Frequent ethical and moral dilemmas add another layer of complexity to the challenges faced by palliative-care workers. These dilemmas often revolve around end-of-life decisions and the management of treatment side effects, intensifying both emotional and psychological stress. These challenges require the palliative-care team to balance medical considerations with respect for the patient's personal values and decisions.[4] Navigating these intricate situations is not just burdening for healthcare professionals; it also deeply affects the patients and their families. This underscores the urgent need for effective stress management tools and support systems tailored to the unique demands of PC.

Some of the several challenges these professionals face in their daily work are:

◆ Patient and Family Caregiver Concordance and Discordance: Decision-making in PC often involves both patients and family caregivers. Discord between them can complicate treatment plans.[5]

◆ Cultural and Social Context: Providing care to patients from diverse backgrounds, including indigenous communities, requires professionals to consider both clinical conditions and cultural sensitivities.[6]

◆ Professional Skills and Expertise: Practitioners rely on their training to discuss end-of-life options, often navigating patient denial of impending death and concerns about legal repercussions.[7]

◆ Unacknowledged Grief Among Healthcare Professionals: Grief that goes unnoticed among healthcare providers can lead to emotional exhaustion, impatience, and burnout.[8]

◆ Communication Challenges: The necessity for effective communication comes with its own set of difficulties, such as discord among family members and the emotional toll of discussing death.[9]

◆ Decision-Making Processes: Choices surrounding end-of-life care are influenced by a myriad of factors, including ethical, sociocultural, religious, political, and economic concerns.[10]

The Emotional Landscape of Palliative-Care Work

Having outlined the primary challenges inherent to PC, it's crucial to delve deeper into the emotional landscape that these complexities often engender.[11]

◆ Communication: Effective communication is a critical skill in PC, as healthcare professionals need to convey sensitive information to patients and their families with empathy and understanding. This may include discussing prognosis, treatment options, and end-of-life preferences. It is essential to strike a balance between honesty and compassion, ensuring that patients and their loved ones are well informed while being emotionally supported. This emotional tightrope can cause stress and requires specialized training and emotional support systems.

◆ Ethical and Legal Dilemmas: Making tough choices about treatments and end-of-life care isn't just complicated, it's emotionally draining. Deciding between medical options and respecting a patient's wishes can often lead to emotional fatigue and ethical distress. Healthcare professionals need a solid ethical foundation and emotional support to navigate these murky waters.

◆ Grieving and Emotional Connection: Grieving the loss of patients is an inevitable part of palliative-care work. Healthcare professionals forge deep connections with their patients and often witness the final stages of their lives. The emotional burden of witnessing suffering and loss can be immense, potentially leading to compassion fatigue or burnout. It is crucial for palliative-care workers to develop healthy coping mechanisms to manage their grief and maintain their emotional well-being.

◆ Work–Life Balance: The long hours and the emotional ups and downs can make it hard for healthcare professionals to maintain a balanced personal life. The emotional weight of their work can carry over into their personal lives, making it crucial for them to have effective stress management strategies.

Addressing these obstacles is fundamental for preserving the well-being of these healthcare workers and ensuring the high-quality care they provide to patients and their families.

Prevalence and Impact of Burnout Among Palliative-Care Workers

Since the World Health Organization officially recognized burnout as a medical diagnosis in 2019, awareness of this syndrome has grown. Although the condition affects various professionals, those in PC stand out with alarmingly high rates. Burnout in this field is characterized by a sense of exhaustion, mental distancing from the job, and a diminished feeling of personal accomplishment, undermining not only the well-being of healthcare providers but also the quality of end-of-life care they offer.[12]

The issue of burnout in PC is a matter of increasing concern, affecting both physicians and nurses. In the United States, the palliative-care community has not been immune to this rising trend. Around 39% of clinicians in the field report feeling burnout, according to a 2020 study. Those most at risk appear to be nonphysician clinicians and younger professionals under age 50. Working long hours, during weekends, and in smaller organizations were other factors compounding their stress.[13] Interestingly, this pattern echoes across the Atlantic. A 2023 survey focusing on UK and Irish palliative-care physicians found similar prevalence rates of burnout.[14]

Nurses, the backbone of PC, are no strangers to burnout either. Around one-fourth of nurses feel emotionally drained, and almost a third report feeling depersonalized in their interactions, affecting their ability to connect meaningfully with patients. These symptoms aren't merely statistics; they translate to a diminished quality of care at a stage in life where patients most need compassion and understanding.[15]

Although the risk factors and prevalence can vary, as shown in a comprehensive review that included an astonishing range of burnout rates from 3% to 66%, one thing remains clear: This is a universal problem.[16] Yet, the same review offers a glimmer of hope, pointing out that specialized palliative-care settings tend to report lower rates compared to general healthcare settings.

Recent scholarly discussion, such as an article by Oldenburger and De Roo, expands our understanding of this issue.[17] They emphasize that individual, social, and organizational dynamics intersect to either exacerbate or mitigate symptoms of burnout among palliative-care professionals.

While understanding the prevalence and impact is foundational, it naturally begs the question: What can be done to address this pervasive issue? As we navigate toward the next section, we will delve into traditional mechanisms of support, as well as pioneering strategies like VR, examining their effectiveness and limitations in mitigating the psychological burden experienced by those in the palliative-care field.

Addressing Burnout and Psychological Burden

Traditional Support Mechanisms: Helpful but Insufficient

Palliative-care workers often deal with complex emotions and situations, requiring them to balance empathy, compassion, and professional boundaries. This emotional labor can lead to burnout, making it essential to develop more tailored and effective support mechanisms.

Although conventional support structures, ranging from supportive supervision and professional development programs to peer support groups and employee assistance programs, have historically been invaluable for mitigating burnout among healthcare professionals, their efficacy has limits. Emerging evidence suggests that interventions involving meditation, communication training, peer-coaching, and art-therapy-based supervision show promise. However, the long-term effectiveness of these approaches remains largely unexplored.[18]

Addressing burnout in palliative-care professionals, a group heavily invested in delivering emotional care and support to patients and their families, requires a nuanced and multi-faceted approach. The complexity arises from the interplay of individual characteristics and environmental influences. Various coping mechanisms have been studied to tackle this issue. Mindfulness techniques, such as mindfulness-based stress reduction (MBSR), have shown promise in alleviating symptoms of burnout. Exercise, too, holds significant potential for stress management and mental well-being. Adequate sleep hygiene is another crucial element for maintaining resilience. Instituting a balanced work–life environment, as opposed to the concept of "total work," allows professionals to engage in activities that bring joy and meaning, which is vital for emotional well-being. Team-based settings and other institutional factors can also provide a supportive role. Despite the helpfulness of these traditional mechanisms, they may not suffice for everyone facing the multidimensional challenges of burnout. This underscores the need for innovative approaches, a subject we delve into in the subsequent section.[19]

By expanding upon traditional support mechanisms and incorporating new approaches, palliative-care workers can be better equipped to manage the emotional and professional challenges they face. This not only helps reduce the prevalence of burnout but also contributes to improved patient care and overall well-being for healthcare professionals in the field.

Immersing in Virtual Reality: A New Frontier in Stress Management

As we explore innovative solutions for enhancing well-being and mitigating burnout in palliative-care workers, the role of technology—specifically, virtual reality—cannot be overlooked. VR marries traditional mindfulness practices with techno-logical innovation, delivering an enriched, immersive mind-fulness experience that has been empirically demonstrated to offer benefits over conventional methods in areas such as mood improvement, sleep quality, and cognitive attention.[20]

The application of VR extends beyond mindfulness; it's a potent tool for healthcare education and mental-health interventions as well. Studies indicate that the immersive nature of VR promotes longer retention of information and enhances learner engagement.[21] This increased level of immersion adds an element of enjoyment to the learning experience, making educational programs more impactful.[22]

What makes VR particularly promising is its capacity to effectively disseminate psychoeducation and relaxation techniques, thereby amplifying its usefulness in mental-health care.[23] Utilizing VR in conjunction with mindfulness training shows promise for combating burnout, a critical concern in palliative-care settings. A comprehensive review by Ma et al. (2023) substantiated these benefits, confirming the effectiveness of immersive VR-based mindfulness practices over traditional approaches.[24]

For palliative-care professionals dealing with the emotional and psychological rigors of their work, practicing mindfulness and emotional management skills in a VR environment could be transformative.[25] This controlled, immersive virtual setting offers healthcare workers a unique opportunity to build the emotional resilience required for their demanding roles, enhancing their overall emotional well-being.

Case Study: Projecte Benestar

Beyond VR Sessions: Proactively Managing Burnout with Mindfulness Training in VR

Although previous studies have shown that VR relaxation can reduce burnout among healthcare workers, our approach takes a more proactive approach to addressing burnout by using VR to teach mindfulness techniques that can be applied anytime and anywhere, empowering health workers to take control of their stress management and self-care beyond the confines of VR sessions.

The Methodology

Our educational program, called *Projecte Benestar*, leverages virtual-reality technology to impart mindfulness and emotional management techniques directly to healthcare professionals, offering an enriched training experience. This initiative not only provides a temporary solution to alleviate stress, but equips healthcare professionals with a tool to help manage stress and prevent burnout from occurring in the first place.

The program consists of eight weekly sessions, each lasting around ten minutes, conducted once a week in an immersive virtual-reality environment. During each session, participants follow the instructions from an audio guide providing explanations on how to use mindfulness and emotion management concepts with the help of the virtual environment to illustrate the techniques.

The simulations are passive scenarios in relaxing environments, allowing participants to observe and experience the virtual environment without the need to interact with it. The program utilizes a range of serene settings, including a sandy beach, a lake, and a Zen garden, among others. These scenes were carefully crafted to be visually captivating and soothing, with some featuring natural sounds like crashing waves or soothing relaxing music.

Addressing VR's Limitations: Standalone and Scalable

Recognizing the limitations of VR, mainly its dependency on high-speed internet and its typically stationary nature, our program incorporates unique features to make it more accessible and practical. The standalone feature of our program, where the sessions are preloaded into the headsets, was highly appreciated by healthcare workers with busy schedules. This allows the program to be integrated effortlessly into the often hectic and unpredictable nature of healthcare work, an essential consideration given the constraints healthcare professionals often face, such as limited time or centers with no Wi-Fi internet connectivity.

It's important to note that the virtual-reality technology we employ serves as a facilitative medium, enhancing the acquisition and practice of mindfulness and emotional management skills. The true potential of these techniques is realized when participants integrate them into their everyday lives. Our program is designed to enable healthcare workers to do precisely that, providing them with not just an immersive learning experience but also with practical skills they can carry into their daily professional and personal lives.

Before diving into the specifics of our case study, it's essential to consider the organizational backdrop against which these initiatives are set. Badalona Serveis Assistencials (BSA) is a comprehensive healthcare service provider located in Badalona, Spain. BSA has been at the forefront of healthcare innovation, continually seeking to integrate cutting-edge technologies and methodologies to improve both patient care and staff well-being. Recognizing the pressing issue of healthcare worker burnout, BSA was quick to sponsor research and pilot programs aimed at this critical concern.

Origin and Evolution of *Projecte Benestar*

Recognizing the emotional toll that healthcare work can have on its professionals, I teamed up with my colleague Nuria Morán Bueno to develop a program aimed at tackling this issue. My own background in family and community medicine, further enriched by work in virtual-reality development, set the technological foundation for the initiative. Nuria, also grounded in family and community medicine, brought a wealth of complementary skills to the project. Her additional training in neurolinguistic programming and mindfulness provided the program with a strong focus on emotional intelligence and stress management.

Our collaboration was fueled by a mutual commitment to combating the rising rates of professional burnout in healthcare. An initial study we conducted at CAP Apenins-Montigalà revealed the efficacy of integrating mindfulness techniques into a virtual-reality framework for reducing stress among healthcare workers. This success prompted us to expand the program, now carefully designed to accommodate healthcare professionals in various roles and settings.

In the initial pilot study at a primary care center, we evaluated 29 of 34 full-time employees, including administrators, clinicians, and support staff. To measure the program's impact, we used the Maslach Burnout Inventory (MBI) for assessing burnout levels and the Utrecht Work Engagement Scale (UWES) for evaluating work engagement. The MBI focuses on emotional exhaustion and depersonalization, while UWES measures how committed and engaged employees are in their work. The data revealed significant improvements, especially for roles with initially high emotional exhaustion and depersonalization scores.

After evaluating the impact of the initial 2022 pilot program, the management team at BSA recognized the transformative potential of our VR-based mindfulness training. This led to a strategic decision to invest in its further refinement and expansion. In 2023, the program was rigorously tested again, this time both at another primary care center and at our specialized intermediate care facility, which houses the Palliative Care Department. Cumulatively, across all the participating groups, we saw an impressive completion rate: 83 out of 90 participants successfully finished the program, resulting in a high retention rate of 95.2%. The minimal attrition was largely due to personal

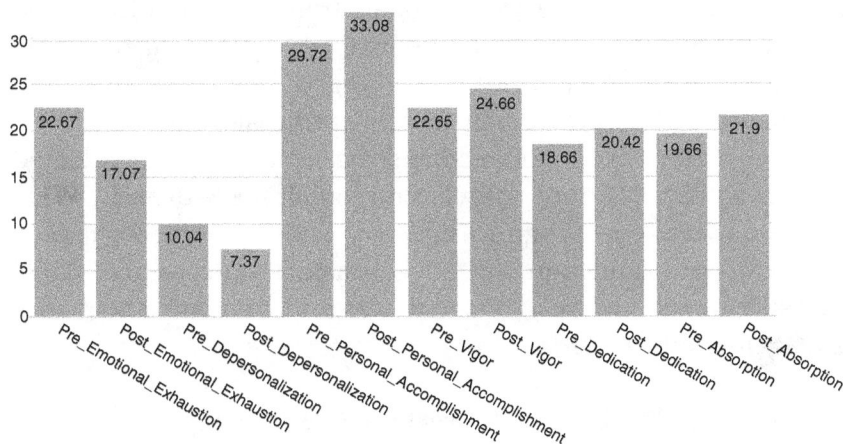

FIGURE 5.2 Summary of pre- and postintervention outcomes among palliative-care professionals participating in VR-based mindfulness training, highlighting significant reductions in burnout levels and improvements in emotional resilience and job engagement.

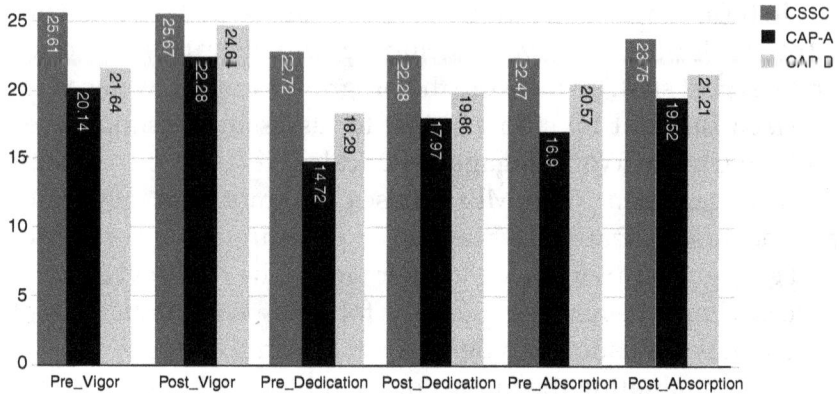

FIGURE 5.3 Summary of the mean scores from the Utrecht Work Engagement Scale (UWES) for the three participant groups prior to and following the intervention.

constraints or time commitments, and notably, there were no dropouts due to discomfort with the VR technology.

Spotlight on Palliative-Care Team Outcomes

The *Projecte Benestar* journey has been especially rewarding in its impact on our palliative-care team, a group grappling daily with high emotional and physical stressors. In a pilot study conducted in 2023 that engaged 41 professionals from this sector, we were not only encouraged by compelling results but also deeply moved by the human stories that emerged.

The retention rate among these 41 professionals was high—36 completed the program, echoing the enthusiasm we've noted in earlier phases of our research. Employing the MBI and UWES, the data was as encouraging as it was quantifiable. Scores related to emotional exhaustion and depersonalization dropped, while measurements around personal accomplishment and work engagement improved.

Making Mindfulness Tangible: A Personal Anecdote

One incident stands out vividly. A palliative-care nurse participating in the program approached me in the hospital corridors one day. With tangible relief, she shared an experience from a particularly challenging shift in the palliative-care ward. She and two other nurses, all part of the program, had taken a mere five-minute break in the control area to practice a technique they'd learned about self-compassion—one I consider critical for healthcare workers like us.

The brief pause helped them reset emotionally, giving them renewed perspective as they returned to their demanding tasks. This real-world application of our program highlights its immediate, practical utility, far beyond statistical validation.

Evolving into Catalysts for a Visionary Approach to Healthcare

Participants, particularly those from the palliative-care team, have now evolved into more than just beneficiaries of the program. What transpired following the launch of *Projecte Benestar* exceeded even my most optimistic expectations. Initially, the mission was bifocal: to raise the emotional resilience of healthcare providers and to explore the potential possibilities of VR within the medical field. However, the outcomes transcended mere program success, starting a wave of creativity and initiative among participants.

Not only did they benefit from the sessions, but they also began to grasp VR's unknown potential. Some of these healthcare professionals, particularly from the palliative-care sector, are now actively developing protocols for clinical research. They aim to use VR to improve quality of life and manage symptoms like anxiety, depression, and pain in their own patients.

It's as if our program has not merely instigated change but also catalyzed a movement. The ripple effects are ongoing, and the collective energy from these healthcare pioneers promises to reshape the contours of patient care for years to come. The exhilarating momentum generated by these frontline healthcare visionaries serves not only as affirmation but also as inspiration to continue pushing the boundaries.

Future Directions and Conclusion

The momentum behind *Projecte Benestar* continues to build. Following the success of our pilot studies and the promising results that emerged from our data analysis, BSA management has given the green light for program expansion. We're now working diligently to introduce our VR-based mindfulness and emotional well-being interventions to six new centers in Badalona. While this phase will not encompass our entire workforce, it's a significant step forward in broadening the program's reach.

The current phase of expansion, while significant, does not yet encompass the remaining members of the palliative-care team who were unable to participate in the pilot studies. Nevertheless, this represents a pivotal interim milestone that signifies the substantial support and investment from BSA's organizational leadership. This endorsement not only validates the efficacy and impact of the program thus far but also serves as a motivational impetus for future research and implementation. The ultimate objective remains: to rigorously extend the program's reach to all healthcare professionals within our organization, including those in specialized sectors such as PC, in forthcoming iterations of the project.

Taking Stock of Achievements and Limitations

Although the *Projecte Benestar* initiative has been a significant stride forward in managing healthcare worker burnout, it's crucial to temper our enthusiasm with a critical examination of the program's limitations. Conducted primarily within the confines of Badalona, Spain, the study's geographical scope remains limited. The immediate positive impact, while compelling, doesn't provide data on long-term effectiveness.

What We've Learned and Where We're Headed

BSA's organizational support has paved the way for an expansion phase, and the ambition doesn't stop there. Collaboration with an external hospital is already in the works to revalidate the program through a study conducted in multiple healthcare centers, where participants switch between receiving the treatment and being in a control group at different times. This new venture will allow for the incorporation of a control group while ensuring that all participants still have access to the program.

Practical Takeaways for What Comes Next

As our program continues to grow, it's critical to keep listening—to the numbers and to the people participating. Here are some of the key lessons we've learned that we think could guide anyone looking to do something similar in the future:

Control Groups and Multicentric Studies: Collaboration with external hospitals could offer new validation layers to the program. This allows for a more robust study design that can include a control group while expanding the program's geographical reach.

Longevity of Impact: Extending the observation period would be instrumental in understanding how long the benefits of the program last and whether they decrease over time.

Broadening Demographics: Diversifying the participant pool by including healthcare professionals from various regions and different tech literacy levels will make the results more generalizable.

Qualitative Approaches: Supplementing the quantitative data with qualitative methods like interviews or focus groups would offer more nuanced insights into participants' lived experiences.

Concluding Remarks on VR and Mindfulness in Healthcare

The progress of *Projecte Benestar* is a shared accomplishment that goes beyond any single vision. It is thanks in part to the considered use of VR technology and the educational contributions of Dr. Nuria Moran, who brings expertise in mindfulness for healthcare workers. This partnership has allowed us to take initial steps toward improving occupational well-being and offers a promising model for building greater resilience in healthcare settings.

VR, as we've seen, isn't merely a dazzling display of technology. It's a catalyst, creating enriched learning environments that are particularly invaluable for professionals navigating the high-stress corridors of healthcare.

By going beyond momentary stress relief to equip healthcare workers with lifelong mindfulness skills, our program aims to enact meaningful, sustainable change. The high success and retention rates, especially among those in the most emotionally taxing roles, suggest that we are on the right track.

We envision our program as a cornerstone for healthcare professionals' well-being, providing them with a toolkit of emotional skills and coping mechanisms that go far beyond the VR headset and into the realities of their challenging work lives.

References

1 World Health Organization. (2020, August 5). "Palliative care." Retrieved from https://www.who.int/news-room/fact-sheets/detail/palliative-care

2 Mæhre, K.S., Bergdahl, E., & Hemberg, J. (2023, November 30). Patients', relatives' and nurses' experiences of palliative care on an advanced care ward in a nursing home setting in Norway. *Nursing Open, 10*(4), 2464–2476. https://doi.org/10.1002/nop2.1503

3 Sekse, R.J.T., Hunskår, I., & Ellingsen, S. (2018, January). The nurse's role in palliative care: A qualitative meta-synthesis. *Journal of Clinical Nursing, 27*(1–2), e21–e38. https://doi.org/10.1111/jocn.13912

4 De Panfilis, L., Di Leo, S., Peruselli, C., Ghirotto, L., & Tanzi, S. (2019, August 9). "I go into crisis when …": Ethics of care and moral dilemmas in palliative care. *BMC Palliative Care, 18*(1), 70. https://doi.org/10.1186/s12904-019-0453-2

5 Mulcahy Symmons, S., Ryan, K., Aoun, S.M., Selman, L.E., Davies, A. Cornally, N., Lombard, J., McQuilllan, R., Guerin, S., O'Leary, N., Connolly, M., Rabbitte, M., Mockler, D., & Foley, G. (2020). Decision-making in palliative care: Patient and family caregiver concordance and discordance-systematic review and narrative synthesis. *BMJ Supportive and Palliative Care*, bmjspcare-2022-003525. Advance online publication. https://doi.org/10.1136/bmjspcare-2022-003525

6 Luna-Meza, A., Godoy-Casasbuenas, N., Calvache, J.A. Díaz-Amado, E., Gempeler Rueda, F.E., Morales, O., Leal, F., Gómez-Restrepo, C., & de Vries, E. (2021). Decision making in the end-of-life

care of patients who are terminally ill with cancer: A qualitative descriptive study with a phenomenological approach from the experience of healthcare workers. *BMC Palliative Care, 20*(1), 76. https://doi.org/10.1186/s12904-021-00768-5May

7 Luna-Meza, A., Godoy-Casasbuenas, N., Calvache, J.A. Díaz-Amado, E., Gempeler Rueda, F.E., Morales, O., Leal, F., Gómez-Restrepo, C., & de Vries, E. (2021). Decision making in the end-of-life care of patients who are terminally ill with cancer: A qualitative descriptive study with a phenomenological approach from the experience of healthcare workers. *BMC Palliative Care, 20*(1), 76. https://doi.org/10.1186/s12904-021-00768-5May

8 Kruczynsk, M. (2015, April 17). Palliative and end-of-life care: Issues, challenges, and possible solutions in the United States. *American Journal of Managed Care*. Retrieved from https://www.ajmc.com/view/palliative-and-end-of-life-care-issues-challenges-and-possible-solutions-in-the-united-states-

9 U.S. Department of Health and Human Services. (n.d.). Making decisions for someone at the end of life. *National Institute on Aging*. Retrieved from https://www.nia.nih.gov/health/making-decisions-someone-end-life; Becker, C., Beck, K., Vincent, A., & Hunziker, S. (2020, September 18). Communication challenges in end-of-life decisions. *Swiss Medical Weekly, 150*, w20351. https://doi.org/10.4414/smw.2020.20351

10 Martins Pereira, S., Fradique, E., and Hernández-Marrero, P. (2018, May 1). End-of-life decision making in palliative care and recommendations of the Council of Europe: Qualitative secondary analysis of interviews and observation field notes. *Journal of Palliative Medicine, 21*(5), 604–615. https://doi.org/10.1089/jpm.2017.0403

11 Martins Pereira, S., Fradique, E., and Hernández-Marrero, P. (2018, May 1). End-of-life decision making in palliative care and recommendations of the Council of Europe: Qualitative secondary analysis of interviews and observation field notes. *Journal of Palliative Medicine, 21*(5), 604–615. https://doi.org/10.1089/jpm.2017.0403; Clayton, M., & Marczak, M. (2022, June 16). Palliative care nurses' experiences of stress, anxiety, and burnout: A thematic synthesis. *Palliative and Supportive Care, 21*(3), 498–514. https://doi.org/10.1017/S147895152200058X

12 World Health Organization. (2023, January), ICD-11 for mortality and morbidity statistics. World Health Organization. Retrieved from https://icd.who.int/browse11/l-m/en#/http://id.who.int/icd/entity/129180281

13 Kamal, A.H., Bull, J.H., Wolf, S.P., Swetz, K.M., Shanafelt, T.D., Ast, K., Kavalieratos, D., & Sinclair, C.T. (2019, November 25). Prevalence and predictors of burnout among hospice and palliative care clinicians. *U.S. Journal of Pain and Symptom Management, 59*(5), e6–e13. https://doi.org/10.1016/j.jpainsymman.2019.11.017

14 Boland, J.W., Kabir, M., Spilg, E.G., Webber, C., Bush, S.H, Murtagh, F., and Lawlor, P.G. (2023, February 15). Over a third of palliative medicine physicians meet burnout criteria: Results from a survey study during the COVID-19 pandemic. *Palliative Medicine, 37*(3), 343–354. https://doi.org/10.1177/02692163231153067

15 Gómez-Urquiza, J.L., Albendín-García, L., Velando-Soriano, A., Ortega-Campos, E., Ramírez-Baena, L., Membrive-Jiménez, M.J., & Suleiman-Martos, N. (2020, October 21). Burnout in palliative care nurses, prevalence and risk factors: A systematic review with meta-analysis. *International Journal of Environmental Research and Public Health, 17*(20), 7672. https://doi.org/10.3390/ijerph17207672. Retrieved from https://www.ncbi.nlm.nih.gov/pmc/articles/PMC7589426/. PMID: 33096682.

16 Dijxhoorn, A.Q., Brom, L., van der Linden, Y.M., Leget, C., & Raijmakers, N.J. (2020, October 16). Prevalence of burnout in healthcare professionals providing palliative care and the effect of interventions to reduce symptoms: A systematic literature review. *Palliative Medicine, 35*(1), 6–26. https://doi.org/10.1177/0269216320956825

17 Oldenburger, E., & De Roo, M.L. (2023, March). Burnout of healthcare professionals in supportive and palliative care: A summary of recent literature. *Current Opinion in Supportive and Palliative Care, 17*(1), 77–83. Retrieved from https://journals.lww.com/co-supportiveandpalliativecare/Abstract/2023/03000/Burnout_of_health care_professionals_in_supportive.12.aspx

18 Dijxhoorn, A.Q., Brom, L., van der Linden, Y.M., Leget, C., & Raijmakers, N.J. (2020, October 16). Prevalence of burnout in healthcare professionals providing palliative care and the effect of interventions to reduce symptoms: A systematic literature review. *Palliative Medicine, 35*(1), 6–26. https://doi.org/10.1177/0269216320956825

19 Horn, D.J., & Johnston, C.B. (2020, May). Burnout and self-care for palliative care practitioners. *Medical Clinics of North America, 104*(3), 561–572. https://doi.org/10.1016/j.mcna.2019.12.007

20 Ma, J., Zhao, D., Xu, N., & Yang, J. (2023). The effectiveness of immersive virtual reality (VR) based mindfulness training on improvement mental-health in adults: A narrative systematic review. *Explore (New York), 19*(3), 310–318. https://doi.org/10.1016/j.explore. 2022.08.001

21 Yang, H., Cai, M., Diao, Y., Liu, R., Liu, L., & Xiang, Q. (2023, January 6). How does interactive virtual reality enhance learning outcomes via emotional experiences? A structural equation modeling approach. *Frontiers in Psychology, 13*, 1081372. https://doi.org/10.3389/ fpsyg.2022.1081372; Moro, C., Štromberga, Z., Raikos, A., & Stirling, A. (2017). The effectiveness of virtual and augmented reality in health sciences and medical anatomy. *Anatomical Sciences Education, 10*(6), 549–559. https://doi.org/10.1002/ase.1696

22 Asad, M.M., Naz, A., Churi, P., & Tahanzadeh, M.M. (2021). Virtual reality as pedagogical tool to enhance experiential learning: A systematic literature review. *Education Research International, 2021*, 1–17, https://doi.org/10.1155/2021/7061623; Barteit, S., Lanfermann, L., Bärnighausen, T., Neuhann, F., & Beiersmann, C. (2021). Augmented, mixed, and virtual reality-based head-mounted devices for medical education: Systematic review. *JMIR Serious Games, 9*(3), e29080, https://doi.org/10.2196/29080; Pascual, K., Fredman, A., Naum, A., Patil, C., & Sikka, N. (2023). Should mindfulness for health care workers go virtual? A mindfulness-based intervention using virtual reality and heart rate variability in the emergency department. *Workplace Health and Safety, 71*(4), 188–194, https://doi. org/10.1177/21650799221123258; Meese, M.M., O'Hagan, E.C., & Chang, T.P. (2021). Healthcare provider stress and virtual reality simulation: A scoping review. Simulation in healthcare. *Journal of the Society for Simulation in Healthcare, 16*(4), 268–274. https://doi .org/10.1097/SIH.0000000000000484

23 Lindner, P., Miloff, A., Hamilton, W., & Carlbring, P. (2019). The potential of consumer-targeted virtual reality relaxation applications: Descriptive usage, uptake and application performance statistics for a first-generation application. *Frontiers in Psychology, 10*, 132,

https://doi.org/10.3389/fpsyg.2019.00132; Oing, T., & Prescott, J. (2018). Implementations of virtual reality for anxiety-related disorders: Systematic review. *JMIR Serious Games, 6*(4), e10965. https://doi.org/10.2196/10965

24 Ma, J., Zhao, D., Xu, N., & Yang, J. (2023). The effectiveness of immersive virtual reality (VR) based mindfulness training on improvement mental-health in adults: A narrative systematic review. *Explore* (New York), *19*(3), 310–318. https://doi.org/10.1016/j.explore.2022.08.001

25 Navarro-Haro, M.V., Modrego-Alarcón, M., Hoffman, H.G., López-Montoyo, A., Navarro-Gil, M., Montero-Marin, J., García-Palacios, A., Borao, L., & García-Campayo, J. (2019). Evaluation of a mindfulness-based intervention with and without virtual reality dialectical behavior therapy®: Mindfulness skills training for the treatment of generalized anxiety disorder in primary care: A pilot study. *Frontiers in Psychology, 10*, 55. https://doi.org/10.3389/fpsyg.2019.00055; Lu, F.I., & Ratnapalan, S. (2023). Burnout interventions for resident physicians: A scoping review of their content, format, and effectiveness. *Archives of Pathology and Laboratory Medicine, 147*(2), 227–235. https://doi.org/10.5858/arpa.2021-0115-EP

6

Creating Awe
Virtual Reality for Palliative and End-of-Life Patients

Teri Yarbrow

In his famous TED talk, Chris Milk, known as the godfather of virtual reality (VR), stated that "Virtual reality is the ultimate empathy machine."[1] For the seriously ill person in palliative and hospice care, it is so much more; it is a device for delivering "awe." When one is facing a terminal illness, VR can be an intervention, an experience of awe that breaks the cycle of depression, fear, and hopelessness.

"Awe is a category of emotion within the spectrum of self-transcendent experiences."[2] Awe is defined by Dacher Keltner, psychologist at the University of California–Berkeley as "the feeling of being in the presence of something vast that transcends your understanding of the world."[3]

In addition, once one experiences awe, there is the need for accommodation: one is never the same. Awe evokes a cognitive shift in perception. The "overview effect" has been described by astronauts looking at planet Earth from space as creating powerful shifts in the way one thinks about Earth and life.

Awe can be experienced in nature, for example, such as during a visit to the Grand Canyon or observing the Northern

DOI: 10.4324/9781032649771-6

Lights. It can also be found in music, art, spiritual and religious experiences, collective group activities, acts of moral beauty, and in everyday miracles of life, like gazing into the eyes of a newborn.

Numerous studies support the potential of VR as a transformative technology, able to induce a personal change.[4] Investigators have used VR to induce awe in laboratories to measure where in the brain awe occurs.[5] "Virtual reality (VR) is a particularly effective mood induction tool for eliciting awe."[6]

Research suggests that awe is a powerful emotion and VR can induce it. Whether a patient is immersed underwater within a pod of dolphins or transported within a shower of light, awe can cause patients to focus on something entirely different than their diagnosis. For someone confined to their bed, immersive VR therapy can deliver an experience that reduces anxiety, relieves pain, enhances quality of life, and can alleviate a crisis of faith by evoking awe and wonder. Teilhard de Chardin wrote that "we are spiritual beings having a human experience."[7] VR can be a potent tool to help patients to reconnect to this inner truth.

Benefits of Awe

The benefits of awe have been increasingly studied since the early 2000s. Neurologists and psychologists have researched and tested the impact of awe on both physical and emotional levels. They have found that experiences of awe can be transformative on both levels. During an experience of awe, bodily functions that are regulated by the vagal nerves in the spinal column have been found to have a calming effect on heart rate and breathing. The nervous system releases the hormone oxytocin that promotes positive feelings like love, nurturing, and bonding. Keltner found that awe can quiet the self-critical voice within by deactivating the default-mode network (DMN) in the cortex. He has written "Awe has a lot of the same neurophysiology of deep contemplation, meditating, reflecting, going on a pilgrimage."[8] Dr. Judith Moskowitz, Northwestern University School of Medicine,

Chicago, reports that "Intentional awe experiences like walks in nature, collective movement, like dance or ceremony, even use of psychedelics improve psychological well-being."[9] The resulting positive emotions can be transformative, and the overall effects are incredible health benefits.

Monroy and Keltner assert that the experience of awe leads to shifts in health and well-being: "Awe engages five processes—shifts in neurophysiology, a diminished focus on the self, increased prosocial relationality, greater social integration, and a heightened sense of meaning—that benefit well-being."[10]

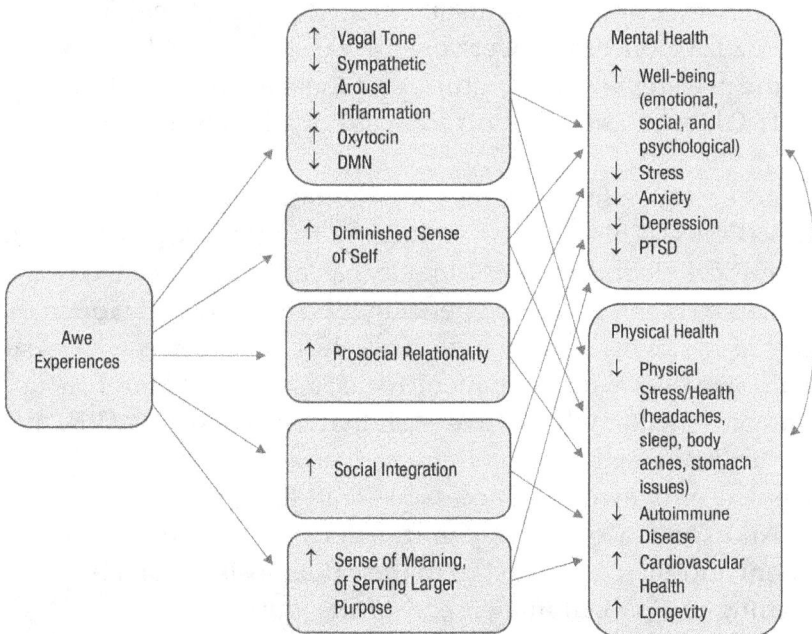

FIGURE 6.1 Model for awe as a pathway to mental and physical health. This model shows that awe experiences will lead to the mediators that will lead to better mental and physical-health outcomes. Note that the relationships between awe experiences and mediators, and mediators and outcomes have been empirically identified; the entire pathways have only recently begun to be tested. One-headed arrows suggest directional relationships, and two-headed arrows suggest bidirectionality.

Note: DMN = default-mode network; PTSD = posttraumatic stress disorder.

Source: Chart courtesy of Dacher Keltner.

Why VR for Palliative and End-of-Life Patients

There is scientific evidence that VR can help distract people from pain. *The Gate Control Theory*, introduced by Ronald Melzack and Patrick Wall in 1965, revolutionized our understanding of pain. The field has expanded since the work of *SnowWorld and Distraction Therapy* by Hunter Hoffman and David Patterson in 1996. Research with VR has expanded greatly since those early years with numerous studies worldwide focusing on the reduction and relief of pain.

Dr. Brennan Spiegel states,

> There has been an exponential rise in the number of peer-reviewed papers that involve XR, VR and healthcare. In 2022 alone, there were over 3,000 studies published in the peer-reviewed literature, and there are now well over 19,000 studies that involve the use of VR in healthcare.[11]

In addition to reducing pain, VR can quiet the default-mode network (DMN). This is the part of the brain that is always watching and critical. Reducing DMN activity can alleviate the anxiety that plagues so many patients. Silencing this inner critic can open the door for an experience of awe. This shift in perception can lead to a flow state, where a patient focuses less on themselves and more on a greater whole. "We posit that Virtual Reality (VR) may help to make self-transcendent and potentially transformative experiences of awe more accessible to individuals."[12]

An experience of awe can transform the life of a palliative patient and their relationship to their diagnosis. It can also bring meaning to a patient in their end-of-life journey.

Case Studies

The following are some amazing case studies from working in palliative care and hospice that illustrate the profound effects of awe in the lives of patients.

Relieving Fear from a Diagnosis

Bernice is an oncology patient in the palliative clinic with extreme fear and anxiety. This is a statement from the admissions administrator in the Steward Center for Palliative Care, Nancy Turcotte:

> To most of us, it was just another clinical day. We had patients show up experiencing no pain. Just a simple follow-up visit, medications refills as needed and out the door they went until their next appointment. Others were in tears. Some were experiencing anxiety and fear. One in particular was feeling all those things and then some. No words could really describe what she was feeling. She simply was and I quote her "a hot mess physically, emotionally and spiritually." This was her first appointment in our palliative care clinic, and she was very emotional. The look on her face reflected no hope, no signs of comfort, fear and pain, so much pain. It was also the first time I was able to introduce VR to clinic patients. I told her that after she saw the clinical staff, that we had a surprise for her. I introduced her to the VR therapist, and I asked her to trust the process and the experience itself.

At the beginning of the VR session, the patient exclaims, "I feel horrible… I have cancer in my back, and it is eating my bones and my insides!... I don't want to die! There's a lot going on. I don't want to lose my life!" Her pain level is a 12 on a scale of 1 to 10 in the preparticipation pain assessment.

The VR session begins with an underwater swim with sea turtles followed by an active enjoyable experience of kayaking in a tropical paradise. It's a distraction from the drama that she's been focusing on. Her attention shifts: "Oh wow! This is wonderful!"

Next Bernice flies over the ocean via VR hang gliding. "I've never experienced anything like this before!" The session ends with a soothing meditation, which focuses her. She exclaims, "I can watch this all day! I feel my pain dropping…. I feel wonderful, I feel fantastic!" Her postparticipation assessment is 0 anxiety, and her pain has dropped to a 3 from 12 on the scale.

When she departs the therapy room, Nancy Turcotte observes:

> I don't know exactly what happened behind closed doors. I don't know exactly which VR experience she did but what I do know is that the patient who walked in there crying, scared, in pain, nervous, hopeless...she came out of there smiling. That smile reflected so much hope. The VR experience was extremely beneficial. She seemed so relieved, just looking at her, everything had changed. She stated she felt so much better. Her walk was different, her demeanor was confident. The VR experience seemed to have a very calming effect on her. She was looking forward to future opportunities to do another VR experience.

Returning to Alignment

Roberta is a Stage 4 cancer patient in constant pain. She suffers from back and lower abdomen pain. When asked how she's feeling and if she is experiencing anxiety due to her pain, she replied, "Yes, I have anxiety. I am aching and have very low energy ... I can't bend over because of the pain... I lost my mother a few months back. It's Christmas time, I'm a minister and I can't help my church ... I'm depressed." She goes through a litany of her symptoms because of her diagnosis. In her preparticipation assessment survey, she describes her pain as 6 on a scale of 1–10. This is her first experience with VR.

Her session begins with a 360 experience of a popular musical on Broadway, *The Circle of Life*. Showing patients something universal, entertaining, and upbeat is a good ice breaker. It is a stirring, almost a gospel, experience for Roberta and she begins to sway with the music.

Next, Roberta experiences an immersive underwater environment. She is encouraged to look above, below, and behind to realize that she surrounded by a pod of 30-plus wild dolphins! The sound is mesmerizing with trance music and dolphin echolocation full of clicks and whistles. VR can transport one in less than 30 seconds because of the brain's capacity to believe a simulation, and as Roberta is transported, she visibly relaxes into the experience. Her breathing slows down.

The final experience is *RadianceVR*. Roberta is encouraged to lean back, look up, and center herself under a pattern of light. Streams begin to fall, engulfing the viewer in a shower of light beams made of 6,500 particles. Minutes later, the light streams form the same pattern at Roberta's feet, and she's encouraged to look down. As above, so below. The music is generously donated for *RadianceVR* by well-known ambient music composer Thom Brennan from a composition called "Silver." The soundtrack inspires one to relax into the experience. Roberta exclaims, "Oh wow! Oh wow! This is so beautiful! It's awesome!" She raises her arms to receive the light and watches *RadianceVR* multiple times. "It's almost like you get energy from it!"

At the end of the session, her postparticipation assessment survey now shows that her pain is at 0 and she has no anxiety. "Absolutely beautiful! I've never experienced anything like it—I could do this every day." Roberta says that she feels good and she's ready to return to her church!

VR evoked a sense of awe for Roberta and shifted her personal crisis of faith. By doing so, Roberta remembered what she already had already known and restored her sense of herself and her purpose. This is an example of the power of VR to transform someone's relationship with a terminal diagnosis.

Hope for an Oncology Patient

Jane, an oncology patient, is 50 years old and has just completed six cycles of chemotherapy. She has a history of Stage IIIC high-grade serous Fallopian tube carcinoma and has tested positive for BRCA1. During the onboarding interview, Jane mentions that she feels fatigued, overwhelmed, and exhausted with her diagnosis. She exclaims, "I feel like I'm burdening my family, like it's my fault." She also mentions that she is feeling "in the dark" and has "lack of motivation to live." Her anxiety is very high, a 10 out of 10 on the preparticipation assessment survey.

Jane's session begins with a journey through Monet's waterlilies at Giverny accompanied by piano music. The colors are vivid as if one is within the painting itself. "Oh my! My lord! Can't believe how real this looks! It's crazy!"

Next Jane experiences an immersive world of abstract light effects and starlight with a soundtrack of soothing music. She begins to cry. "Oh, this is so good! Takes your mind off things. Very peaceful."

Jane enters an immersive guided meditation. Her breathing slows and her body relaxes. "I feel like I can breathe again! I am not selfish for breathing."

At the end of the experiences, Jane's anxiety is now a level 4 out of 10. Her posture has improved, and she is no longer slumped over, hidden in her layers of clothes. "I wish I could have had VR during my chemo infusions. I've had to endure many treatments. It would have made a world of difference! I would have been there, but *not there!*"

By joining the VR trial, her mood has dramatically changed as well as her vision and outlook on her life. She remarks that she can let go of the shame and self-blame she carries because of her diagnosis. "I feel hopeful." This is an example of the power of VR to transform a patient's sense of self.

Awesome Power of Presence through Music

Bill is a Hospice patient and former gospel musician. He watches gospel music on his phone's YouTube app all day. He loves to share videos of live music performances online and is very excited to show them to volunteers, nurses, and staff. Having had a debilitating stroke, he has difficulty speaking; however, he communicates that when he was younger, he played piano and, obviously, loves music.

Bill's session begins with live music experiences in VR. It is clear that he is enjoying them, and mutters, "Cool!" Taking off the headset, he then shows the therapist one of his favorites on his phone.

Next, he is shown the same performance, his favorite that he was watching on his phone, although now he encounters it in VR. Once he enters the experience, he lights up! He sways with the music and hum-sings along. He is watching a performance of himself when he was younger playing in a gospel band! The performance is in a large room filled with joy, an auditorium full of people, dancing and clapping and singing along. He is playing with all of his band mates, smiling and being with each other once again. Bill is overwhelmed, raises his hands, and tears roll down his cheeks!

Research suggests that music can improve mood and well-being. Studies have shown that when people listen to music it helps them return to themselves in an improved way.

> Listening to and performing music reactivates areas of the brain associated with memory, reasoning, speech, emotion, and reward. Two recent studies—one in the United States and the other in Japan—found that music doesn't just help us retrieve stored memories, it also helps us lay down new ones.[13]

Watching himself in VR transports Bill back into one of his own performances on stage and evokes a sense awe. He is ecstatic

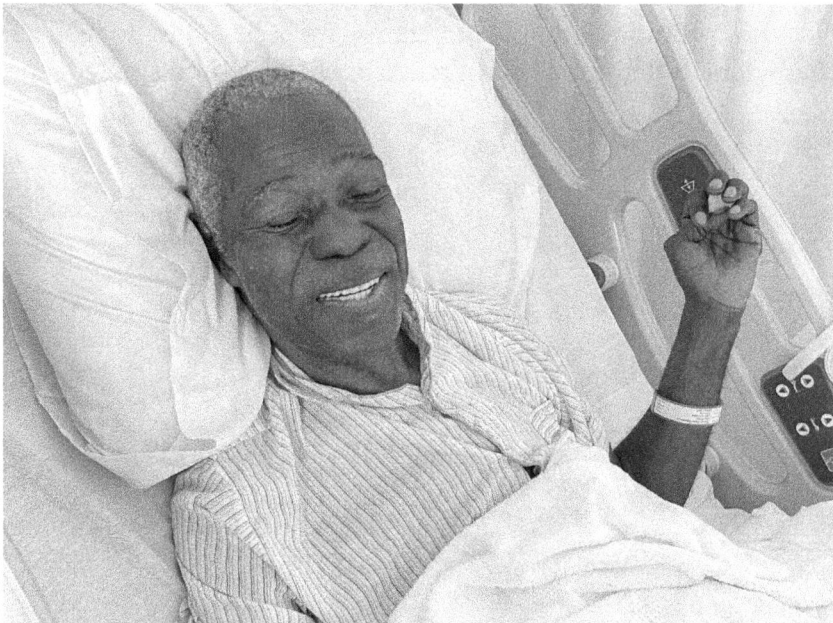

FIGURE 6.2 Bill's response to watching his performance in VR.

and cries tears of joy. This is an example of the power of VR to transform someone's end-of-life experience.

Looking Beyond the Diagnosis

Tom is a Stage 4 cancer patient who suffers from anxiety about his terminal diagnosis. He is communicative about preparing for his ultimate death. He discussed several philosophies about what happens at the moment of death: Buddhism, traditional Western religions, and other modern schools of thought. However, his anxiety prevents him from relaxing and enjoying his life, and he complains of sleeplessness.

During his first session with VR, he watched several contemplative experiences. He was transported through VR to fantasy worlds with soothing sounds and guided meditations.

> Focus on the light...
> breathe in with the particles,
> hold it… now exhale.
> Time your breath with the flow.[14]

He was prompted to play a game with his eyes to control characters in flight. His body relaxed, his breathing slowed, and

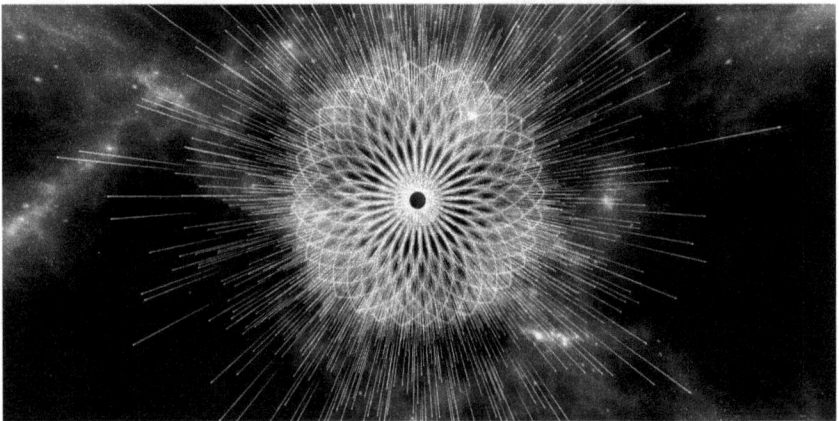

FIGURE 6.3 Radiance VR image.
Source: Created by Teri Yarbrow, Max Almy, and Josephine Leong.

he was noticeably calmer. Tom exclaims, "This is so cool! I've never done anything like this before! I feel like I'm there!"

The session ended with experiencing an immersive shower of light, which Tom watched continuously three times. At the end of the session, his postparticipation assessment survey shows that his anxiety is at 0! He exclaims, "This must be what a near death experience is like!... If this is what death is like, I'm not afraid to die!"

VR evoked a sense of awe for this patient. It was transcendent and transformational. He was able to look beyond his diagnosis and his fear. VR helped Tom get in touch with his spirituality. This is an example of the power of VR to transform someone's relationship with their mortality.

Reclaiming Her Life

Frida, a 50-year-old mother, photographer, and ceramicist has just been diagnosed with progressive spondyloarthritis. Growing stiffer and unable to do everyday tasks because crippling joint pain is overwhelming and debilitating, Frida suffers from depression, fear, and anxiety with her prognosis and the choice of options. She is experiencing confusion on which doctor's advice to take. One option is a chemo protocol with hair loss and other side effects, a second option is to not take the medication that makes her feel sick, and she questions the accuracy of her diagnosis. A third option is to just make lifestyle changes. Her confusion is overwhelming, and her anxiety is off the scale at the beginning of her first session. She complains of dull, achy gnawing pain in her groin and her shoulder.

During her first VR session, she begins to cry as a flood of memories pours in during immersive music. She recalls times of joy with her family and eases into the experience as her breathing slows.

Next Frida experiences Immanence VR, a stirring reflection on the tree of life and seasons created solely in VR in a painterly style. The music is upbeat and inspirational, and the environments are pulsing with energy. Her body language relaxes as she looks all around her and it's apparent that she's thoroughly enjoying the immersion. She watches it numerous times and exclaims, "That's amazing! So cool, I feel like I'm a part of it!"

The session ends with a contemplative experience that helps Frida return to herself, and she makes a positive decision to work with her doctor and implement lifestyle changes. Her anxiety and confusion are now 0 on her postparticipation assessment survey.

At the beginning of the session, she complained of too many voices in her head; now she feels clearly able to hear her own voice and quiet the noise inside.

Frida experienced a profound shift in her point of view; she realized that her life is bigger than her diagnosis, that she has many choices, and she can make them daily. The session evoked a sense of awe, and she has returned to her practice of meditation, yoga, and ceramics.

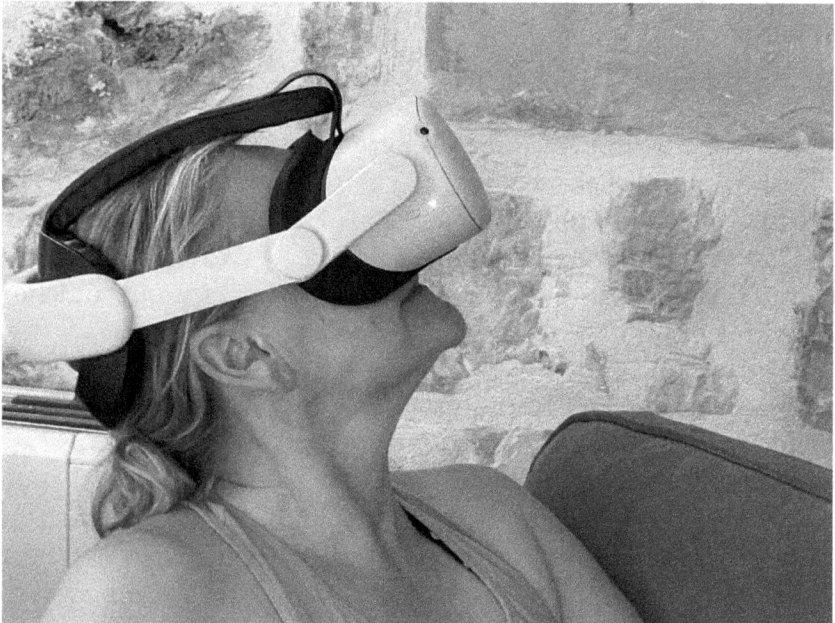

FIGURE 6.4 Frida experiencing VR.

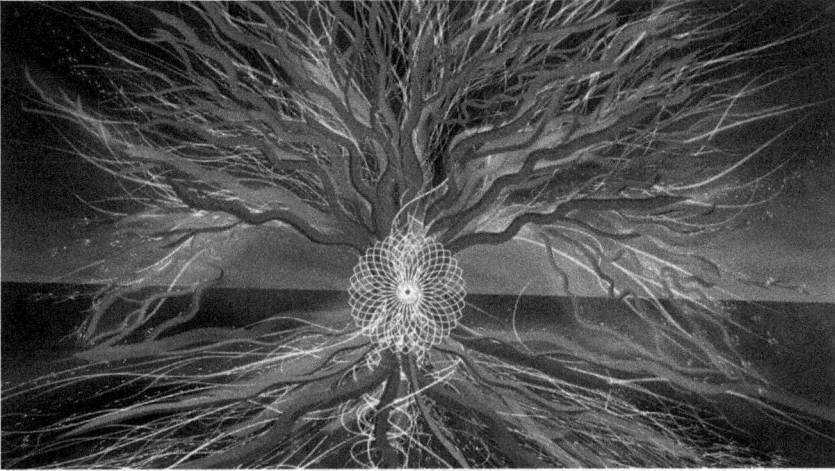

FIGURE 6.5 Immanence VR, Teri Yarbrow and Max Almy. Programming: Amir Ahmadi, 3D Animation: Andy Atkins.

Bart: Making Peace with Terminal Diagnosis

Bart suffers from idiopathic pulmonary fibrosis. He has been given a prognosis of three years to live, however, he is in year four! His lungs are at 43% capacity with a recent 15% drop. Bart experiences anxiety from not being able to breathe and the "knowledge that you're going to die."

Bart, a talented artist, is shown immersive Monet waterlilies at Giverny as his first experience with VR. Instantly he is transported into three-dimensional impressionistic paint strokes. He remarks, "The colors are amazing! Wow! The water is rippling... This is a show unto its own!" He begins to relax into the session, which includes experiences that are playful and gently ease him into the experience to get him beyond the initial shock of the 360-degree immersive worlds. As he swims underwater and explores reefs, he exclaims, "Wow, this is so playful!"

Next is a meditation experience that is procedurally generated based on a patient's emotional state. "Look into the light and time your breath with the flow" is a prompt from the meditation.[15]

This is challenging for Bart because his breathing is shallow. He is able to continue with the contemplation but has difficulty with any of the breath work. Next, he is shown a visual meditation, Immanence, that is based on the tree of life and the life cycles of nature. Energy particles flow in and out of an arche-typal tree and there's a mycelium network below the roots pulsing with life. It's a metaphor for the enduring power of nature. Bart connects deeply with this experience and watches it eight times: "So amazing! It's beautiful. I feel so excited … the mandalas! Incredible experience of the tree of life."

The session concludes with Radiance VR, which invites Bart into an immersive shower of light. He watches it four times and felt "the light was hitting right in my chest where I need help!" Hours after the session and into the next day, he expressed that "he could return to the vision, the state that the VR had created for him." Virtual reality evoked a sense of awe and well-being for Bart, and he plans to continue exploring immersive programs that will enable him to draw in VR.

His caregiver and life partner, Hannah, had a profound experience as well. Hannah is a psychotherapist and very open

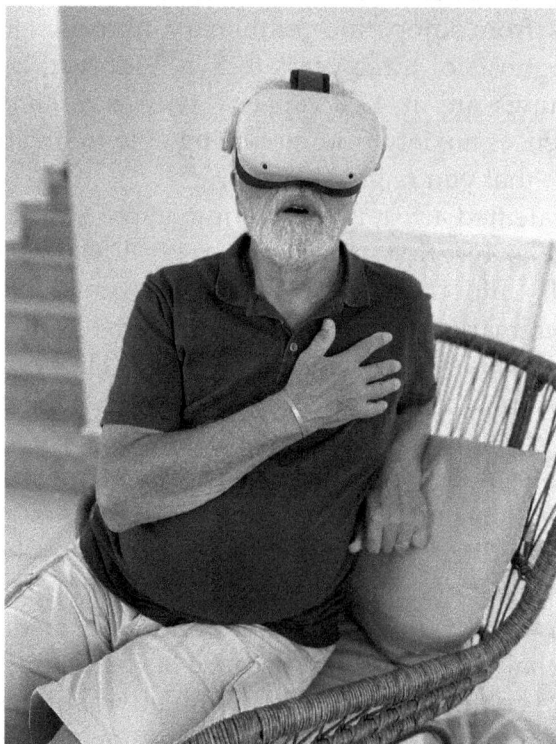

FIGURE 6.6 Bart experiencing the light from VR in his chest.

to alternative treatments. This is her first time in VR. She watched Radiance VR six times and exclaimed,

> Oh! The flower of life! I'm going through the tunnel to God! It's wonderful... If you die, this must be the feeling you have ... I love it! Like taking a drug, being in a psychedelic state. Beautiful! Wow... My throat chakra is beating! I have a blockage in my throat, my weak spot, and I can feel the light there!

The day after the session, Hannah remarked, "We can still put ourselves in the same vision and feeling! [It] raises the level of consciousness. That is great."

VR and Transformation

Palliative care and hospice can be a profound time in the life of a patient and their family, and it can be vehicle for awakening. Elizabeth Kuebler-Ross, a Swiss-American psychiatrist, researched the end-of-life experience and identified five stages associated with grief in her book *On Death and Dying*. These stages have been defined as denial, anger, bargaining, depression, and acceptance. Using VR with palliative and end-of-patients has led to the observance of a further step: transformation.

Figure 6.7 shows how diagnosis can be a life-changing event.

In a famous lecture, Ram Dass, American spiritual teacher and psychologist, wrote, "Each of us contains a being that doesn't die and a being that does die."

This is an existential concept: how does a patient with a terminal illness come to terms with this awareness?

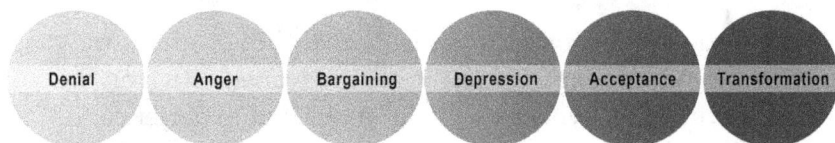

FIGURE 6.7 Diagnosis can be a life-changing event.

Serious illness is an opportunity for spiritual awakening. Studies suggest that awe from a spiritual experience can improve mental and physical health, promote well-being, and instill a sense of meaning.[16]

Dale Borglum, with Ram Dass and Stephen Levine, founded the conscious dying movement in the West. He was the executive director of the Living/Dying Project. In an interview on livingdying.org, he exclaims,

> Whether it is the death of someone deeply loved or leaving behind one's own body, or being in attendance during someone's dying, the dying process is potentially the most direct and immediate opportunity for spiritual awakening of an entire lifetime.[17]

Awe can also evoke feelings of spirituality, a sense of connection to the divine. Awe is central to the mystical experience that people often deem "spiritual." This experience is cultivated by religious ritual, ceremony, and practice (for example, prayer, chanting, or sacred music). In fact, awe is a key item in the most widely used measure of mysticism.[18] Awe, as William James suggested, is core to the religious experience.[19]

Oftentimes, palliative and hospice patients are depressed, they ruminate, obsess, or focus on diagnosis and the imminence of death. VR can be an intervention into this cycle and a vehicle for inducing awe. VR has also been described as a "cyberdelic" digital technology combined with properties of mind expansive psychedelics.[20] Studies indicate that psychedelics and VR are used in analogous ways to alter sensory experience and evoke awe.[21] VR as a cyberdelic can evoke psychedelic imagery and ego dissolution. It can also bring about a change in perception and an altered state of consciousness.

> Cyberdelic technologies are fast emerging as an entirely new type of experience. Whilst psychedelics can be unpredictable, cyberdelics offer a curated experience for an altered state one that can be explored in a completely

safe and controlled way. It is a term used to describe the immersion in cyberspace as a psychedelic experience.[22]

VR can be an agent for awakening, as it gets patients into the moment. As a medium that induces presence, the sense of being there, it helps patients to remember who they are. A deep immersion can remind a patient of things they enjoy and people they love. VR can transport patients to places they have visited or items on their bucket list that they want to visit in the final chapter of their life. It has the potential to change the patient experience from ruminating over their condition. Immersion can break the cycle of pain and depression. This can improve the quality of life for patients and bring about a change in consciousness.

By using VR to induce awe, it can shift a patient's eyes off their diagnosis and provoke a profound change. Patients become aware that there is so much more than their identification with the illness. The moment the patient takes their eyes off their diagnosis, there can be transformation. A patient can experience a connection to something greater than themselves, a transformation of their view of their own mortality, and a heightened sense of meaning in their life.

References

1 Milk, C. (2015). How virtual reality can create the ultimate empathy machine. TED. Retrieved from https://www.ted.com/talks/chris_milk_how_virtual_reality_can_create_the_ultimate_empathy_machine?language=en

2 Quisnel, D., & Reicke, B.E. (2018, November 8). Are you awed yet? How virtual reality gives us awe and goosebumps. *Frontiers in Psychology, 9: 1.*

3 Keltner, D. (2023). *Awe, The science of everyday wonder and how it can transform your life.* New York: Penguin.

4 Chirico, A., Yaden, D.B., Riva, G., & Gaggioli, A. (2016, November). The potential of virtual reality for the investigation of awe. *Frontiers in Psychology, 8: 5.*

5 Chirico, A., Cipresso, P., Yaden, D.B., Biassoni, F, Riva, G., & Gaggioli, A. (2017, April 27). Effectiveness of immersive videos in inducing awe: An experimental study. *Nature, Scientific Reports.* https://doi.org/10.1038/s41598-017-01242-0

6 Chirico, A., Yaden, D.B., Riva, G., & Gaggioli, A. (2016, November). The potential of virtual reality for the investigation of awe. *Frontiers in Psychology, 8*: 1.

7 Pierre Teilhard de Chardin. (1993). In Furey, R.J. (1993), *The joy of kindness.* Chestnut Ridge, NY: Crossroad.

8 Reese, H. (2023, January 3). How a bit of awe can improve your health. *New York Times.*

9 Reese, H. (2023, January 3). How a bit of awe can improve your health. *New York Times.*

10 Monroy, M., & Keltner, D. (2023). Awe as a pathway to mental and physical health. *Perspectives on Psychological Science, 18*(2) 309–320. https://doi.org.10.1177/17456916221094856

11 Los Angeles, Apr10, 2023 vMed23: How virtual reality is transforming medicine. *Cedars-Sinai Organization.* Retrieved from https%3A%2F%2Fwww.cedars-sinai.org%2Fnewsroom%2Fvmed23-how-virtual-reality-is-transforming-medicine%2F

12 Quesnel, D., & Riecke, B. (2018, November 8). Are you awed yet? How virtual reality gives us awe and goosebumps. *Frontiers in Psychology, 9*: 1.

13 Fabiny, A. (2015, February 14). Music can boost memory and mood. *Harvard Women's Health Watch.*

14 Daily flow meditation. *Tripp VR.* Retrieved from https://www.tripp.com.

15 Daily flow meditation. *Tripp VR.* Retrieved from https://www.tripp.com.

16 Monroy, M., & Keltner, D. (2023). Awe as a pathway to mental and physical health. *Perspectives on Psychological Science, 18*(2), 309–320. https://doi.org/10.1177/17456916221094856

17 Rubin, H.J. (1983, January). Living with dying: An interview with Dale Borglum. *Sun Magazine.*

18 Hood, R.W. (1975). The construction and preliminary validation of a measure of reported mystical experience. *Journal for the Scientific Study of Religion, 14*(1), Article 29.

19 Yaden D.B., Zhao Y., Peng K., Newberg A.B. (2020). *Rituals and practices in world religions* (Vol. 5). Springer. Retrieved from http://link.springer.com/10.1007/978-3-030–27953-0

20 Spiegel, B. (2020). *VRx: How virtual therapeutics will revolutionize medicine*. New York: Basic Books.

21 Aday, J.S., Davoli, C.C., & Bloesch, E.K. (2020 August 14). Psychedelics and virtual reality: Parallels and applications. *Therapeutic Advances in Psychopharmacology*. https://doi.org/10.1177/2045125320948356

22 Kumar, V. (2022, June 6). Cyberdelic is the hottest topic in the VR town. *Industry Wired*. Retrieved from https://industrywired.com/cyberdelic-is-the-hottest-topic-in-the-vr-town/

7

The Art of Immersive Storytelling with Bio-Data

Sarah Hill

In 2009, Rob Walker and Joshua Glenn demonstrated the power of story and how it enhances an otherwise regular object into something with greater subjective value. They purchased a variety of items at garage sales and thrift stores. A writer was paired with each trinket. Those writers created fictional stories about each item. The items were put up for sale on eBay. The listing made clear that the stories were fake. The winning bidders received the trinkets along with the stories. In the end, the project designers spent just $128 on the items from thrift stores and garage sales. But with stories attached, those same items sold for more than $3,600!

Stories have the power to enhance not only subjective value of thrift store items but when paired with bio- or neurofeedback, immersive stories also provide a healing glimpse inside ourselves.

Seeing Your Feelings

Do you struggle with traditional meditation? For some people, even after years of practice, when they close their eyes to

DOI: 10.4324/9781032649771-7

meditate, they "see" nothing and wonder, "Am I doing this right?" When you flex your arm muscle, you see your bicep moving up and down. But when you meditate, it's difficult for the average person to know whether their mind is relaxed because they can't see it. How are you supposed to learn to control what you can't *see*? Immersive stories paired with bio-data like the electroencephalogram (EEG), heart rate, blood pressure, and skin conductance enable you to see your feelings and get feedback on your mind's or heart's state. With new tools like generative artificial intelligence (AI), that bio-data can not only create feedback inside immersive stories but it can also *create* new stories altogether.

Take, for instance, a Healium story where you use a magic wand to spawn different spirit animals based off of your EEG or heart rate. If your mind is calm, your EEG data is transformed into a dove, wolf, or jaguar or an entirely new animal altogether. Your body's energy is actually creating that asset!

Stories are how we learn, how we make sense of the world. Stories have the have the ability to hurt…and heal.

Digital Nutrition and Negative Fiber

For example, consider the constant stream of news on television and online. Whether it is the aftermath of the global pandemic or coverage of war, what you consume in the media also impacts your mental health. It's important to note that just as you need to take care of your *physical* health through a nutritious diet, you also need to take care of your *mental* health by minding how your media diet is affecting your stress. Extended reality (XR) is a powerful media detox for your mind because it tricks your brain into thinking you're somewhere else.

Research on the effects of news media in the past decades have shown a distinct impact on how one views and responds to the world. Communication researchers have studied "cultivation theory" (2015) among television viewers and now (2023) those heavily active on social media.[1]

Cultivation theory asserts that those who watch television for many hours will adopt a view of the world that mirrors what they watch on television. For those who watch the news constantly, it may be a heightening view of a "scary world," with rampant crime and violence, social turbulence, or lately, a very bleak and hopeless future because of the current coronavirus pandemic.

Also, there's a term in journalism: "If it bleeds, it leads": Those stories that have direct impact in terms of numbers of those affected or impacted within a society will be seen as the top story, and this is especially true if the story involves bloody, violent, or deadly action.

As a former news broadcaster for more than two decades, the poor media diet that I consumed daily ultimately made me sick. Ruminating thoughts led to insomnia and my body backfired with panic attacks. I now use XR to quiet my mind and increase my focus as a media detox.

Obviously, global news events are the top stories but in a constant media stream on TV and online, the "emotionalizing" of stories, almost trying to find the new angle or latest victim, can affect psychological health.[2]

The groundbreaking documentary *Social Dilemma* illustrates the impact of poor digital nutrition and mental-health concerns making the argument that the technology that connects us can also manipulate us.[3]

Your Brain on Stress

For your brain, stress is stress, no matter if you watch the news or are being chased by a lion. A section of your brain called the amygdala is designed to scan for danger or threats in the environment. According to Dr. Jeff Tarrant, director of the NeuroMeditation Institute[4] and chief scientist for Healium XR, when something is seen as a potential danger, that part of the brain activates the body's stress response and will remain "on" until the threat is resolved.[5]

"When we continually take in more 'evidence' of the threat through news and social media it reinforces the threat response," said Dr. Tarrant. "On the other hand, if you can send the nervous system signals that it is safe, it can begin to relax the hyper-vigilance, nervousness, and worry that comes with an over aroused amygdala."

Does that mean you have to stop watching the news? No. But you need to eat some positive media fiber. That's where virtual reality (VR) and augmented reality (AR) or immersive media comes in.

You need to eat good food and get plenty of exercise and rest to be physically healthy. In the same way, you can think of your media consumption as "food" for your mind.

I like to think of inspirational broadcasts and podcasts, good music, and being out in nature as ways to wash out the negative fiber in my digital diet.

If you can't make it outside and only have a few minutes, immersive media experiences can also balance out the negative fiber from the constant media.[6]

But it's a balance.

If you eat too much dessert, you will get sick. It's the same with the news media: We just can't help listening to the latest

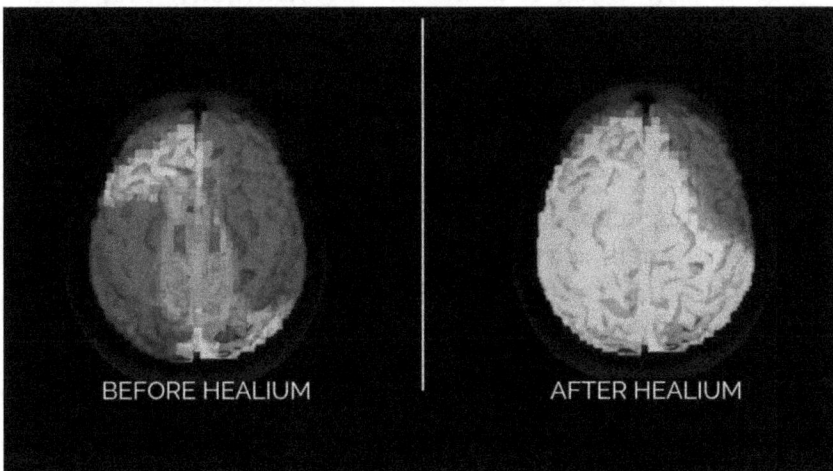

BEFORE HEALIUM | AFTER HEALIUM

FIGURE 7.1 (Red) = High beta activity in the brain of a firefighter immediately before virtual reality and four minutes after as captured with a 20-electrode EEG cap. The fast activity in the brain was significantly reduced from this immersive media therapy.

scandal—but one bite and we're tempted to binge watch for the next ambulance-chasing story.

When you're watching the news or trying to get the latest updates online, just remember two things: Your feelings have power. You have the ability to use drugless, nonharmful coping mechanisms like VR and AR to downshift your nervous system and relieve your stress. There are more than 900 published studies on the therapeutic use cases of VR and AR to reduce anxiety,[7] improve mood,[8] and even increase engagement rates[9] compared to 2D media.

One of the things I'm fascinated with is the ability of VR and AR to shift brain patterns away from the stress response. To better understand how this happens, we've spent years studying how the brain responds to immersive media. According to Dr. Jeff Tarrant on how XR impacts the brain, "Every time a brain cell fires, there is an accompanying electrical impulse. These individual impulses are far too small to be read by any standard equipment. However, because our brain is composed of hundreds of thousands of neurons firing hundreds of times per second and in communication with each other, we can pick up any organized patterns that emerge."

Essentially, when neurons fire in synchrony, they create bursts of electrical activity. These symphonies of neuronal firing are read by sensors placed on the scalp. Because there is so much electrical activity happening at any particular moment, the signal we receive is a bit on the messy side. It's messy because it's essentially a collection of everything occurring at any particular moment in one region. This pattern is the raw EEG and its signal looks something like this:

Figure 7.2 is a screen-capture of a 19-channel EEG signal. Essentially, this recording is examining 19 locations on the scalp simultaneously.

This is what we see on the scanners in the background of medical TV shows and what most people imagine when they think of brainwaves. However, this group of squiggly lines doesn't mean much unless you are a neurologist or an EEG technician.

These squiggly lines are very useful in a hospital setting when looking for gross abnormalities such as a seizure. However, if we

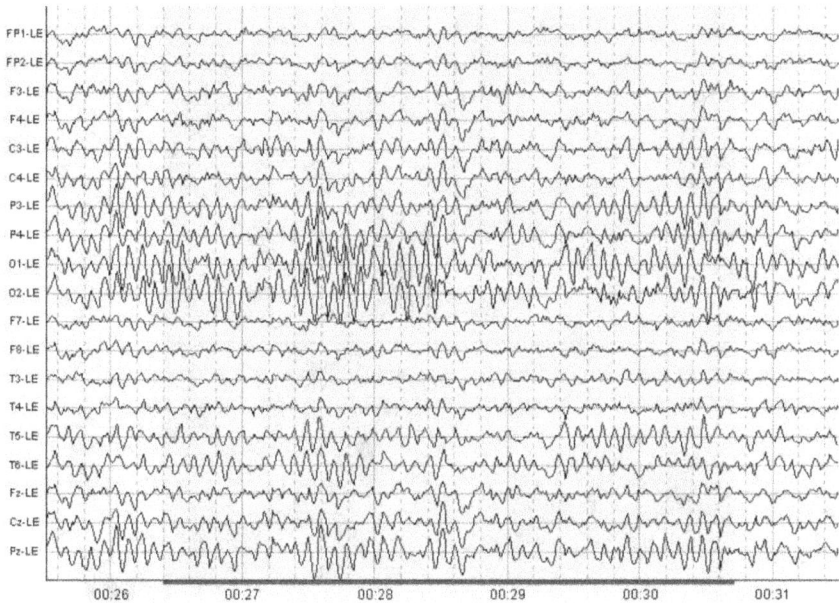

FIGURE 7.2 Screen-capture of a 19-channel EEG signal.

are wanting to look at more subtle changes in consciousness, the raw signal leaves much to be desired.

Lucky for us, techniques have been developed to take a raw EEG recording, like the one in Figure 7.2, and filter it, allowing us to see all of the different frequencies contained within each of those 19 channels. This deserves a bit of an explanation.

Brainwaves, just like any electrical signal, can be described in terms of their frequency and amplitude. Frequency refers to how many repetitions there are of the wave within a second of time, usually referred to as cycles per second (cps) and reported as Hertz (Hz).

If the image in Figure 7.3 represents one second of time and there are two cycles occurring (each peak to peak is considered one cycle), we would describe this as 2 Hz activity. At any given moment, the brain is producing frequencies from as slow as you can measure (below 1 Hz) to an unknown speed (we are still trying to figure this out). However, the vast majority of brainwaves occur between 1 and 50 Hz. Consequently, brainwaves in this range are nearly always the focus of brainwave analyses.

The other dimension of electrical activity that is important to understand relates to power. If speed is measured in hertz and relates to how many repetitions occur in a second of time, power

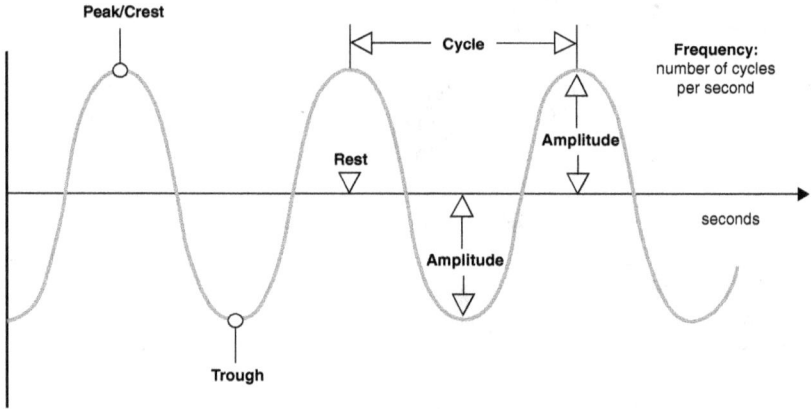

FIGURE 7.3 Brainwave frequency diagram.

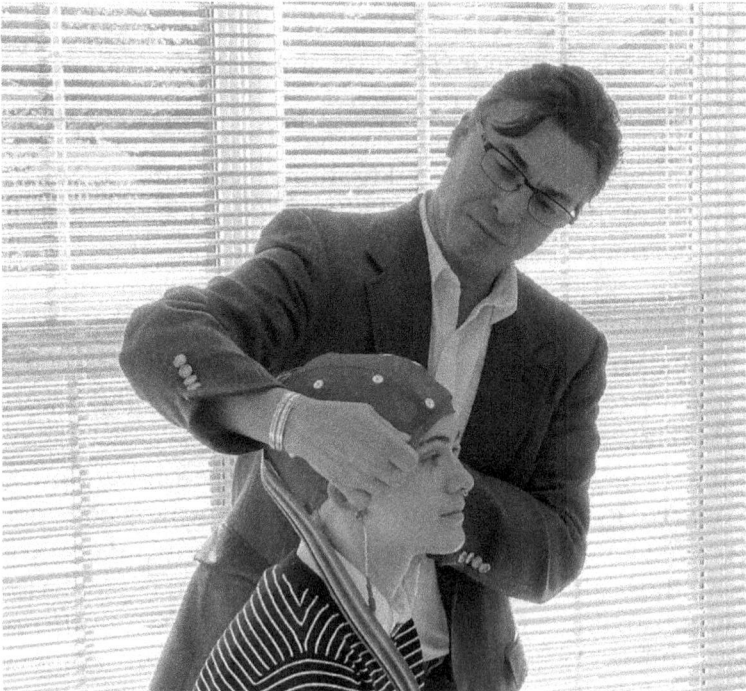

FIGURE 7.4 EEG sensor cap used to measure brainwaves.

is measured in microvolts and measures how big the waveform is. It is essentially a calculation of the average peak to trough of the electrical signal. On the "brainwave metrics" diagram, the vertical (y) axis displays the range of power.

In nonhospital settings, the EEG sample is processed through a mathematical formula (fast Fourier transform, FFT) that separates the various frequencies within the raw signal and averages the power of each frequency, giving you a concrete measurement of "how much" activity is happening at different frequencies.

At any given moment, at any point on the surface of the brain, you will find electrical activity of every frequency we can measure, from the very slow (1–2 Hz) to the very fast (100 Hz). That is a bit overwhelming to consider and is typically simplified by creating clusters of frequencies that many people have at least heard of, including delta, theta, alpha, and beta.

Brainwave Bands

Brainwave bands are simply clusters of frequencies that are lumped together based loosely on their shape and function. Different researchers, neurofeedback companies, and clinicians define these EEG bands slightly differently. The BrainLink Lite headband,[10] one of the headbands used with Healium, uses the following categories:

Delta (0.5–2.75 Hz)
Theta (3.5–6.75 Hz)
Low Alpha (7.5–9.25 Hz)
High Alpha (10–11.75 Hz)
Low Beta (13–16.75 Hz)
High Beta (18–29.75 Hz)
Low Gamma (31–39.75 Hz)
Mid Gamma (41–49.75 Hz)

Delta Waves
Delta waves (0.5–2.5 Hz) are the slowest brainwaves. When they are dominant, the person in question is probably unconscious.

Just to be clear, we always have delta activity, but when it increases significantly, it will be very difficult (if not impossible) to maintain any sort of alert consciousness. When this frequency is dominant, the brain is involved in resting and regeneration. Think about what is happening during deep sleep. You might also see heightened delta activity in areas of the brain that have been damaged in some way. Again, it is the brain's way of shutting things down for repair.

Theta Waves

Theta waves (3.5–6.75 Hz) are obviously a bit faster than delta but still very slow. These brainwaves tend to increase while retrieving certain types of memories, in moments of creativity, and during the "twilight state" that we experience just before falling asleep. Theta waves are often associated with the subconscious. As such, this is generally the place that people shift toward during a hypnotic state—a state that is more open, creative, and suggestible. This also happens to be the dominant frequency for young children.

Low Alpha Waves

Low alpha waves (7.5–9.25 Hz) refer to the frequency range rather than the amplitude of the waves when used in this way. To minimize confusion, this band is sometimes referred to as Alpha1. Alpha is like our neutral, our idling speed. Low alpha is generally associated with being relaxed and internally focused. For this reason, it is generally associated with states of meditation, similar to transcendental meditation or Zen.

High Alpha Waves

High alpha waves (10–11.75 Hz) are often referred to as Alpha2 and are associated with a mental state of open awareness or quiet readiness. This implies that someone is capable of responding to a wide range of changes in the environment. In peak performance training, this state is associated with fast reflexes and accurate responses. This state may be a component of being in "the zone" or a flow state.

Low Beta Waves

Low beta waves (13–16.75 Hz) are observed in the sensorimotor cortex, and are referred to as the sensorimotor rhythm (SMR). They are connected to reduced attention to sensory input and decreased motor activity. It can be thought of as mentally alert without action or "reflecting before acting." When this pattern is observed in other areas of the brain, it is referred to as low beta or Beta1. This band often increases during problem solving.

High Beta Waves

High beta waves (18–29.75 Hz) represent a frequency range that is often elevated during anxiety, worry, or rumination or in connection with emotional intensity. This band can also increase during productive cognitive engagement or working too hard (over-efforting).

Low Gamma Waves

Low gamma waves (31–39.75 Hz) are sometimes considered another range of high beta rather than gamma. These frequencies often demonstrate high amplitudes in persons who are worried, ruminating, feeling "stressed out," or are hypervigilant.

Mid-Gamma waves

Mid-gamma waves (41–49.75 Hz) represent a range of brain waves that are obviously very fast. They are generally at the top of the range that you will see in any research or brain training. Increases in mid-gamma waves are associated with a very sharp focus and feelings of creativity, insight, and being energized. Bursts of this frequency are often seen during high-level information processing or when various parts of the brain are working together to integrate information. Unlike beta forms of processing, mid-gamma activation is often associated with a more effortless, easy form of understanding, such as we might see during an "aha" moment—effortless insight.

Hopefully, you can begin to see how and why the fluctuations in different brain waves can often tell us something about the person's state of consciousness *and* how certain patterns—such

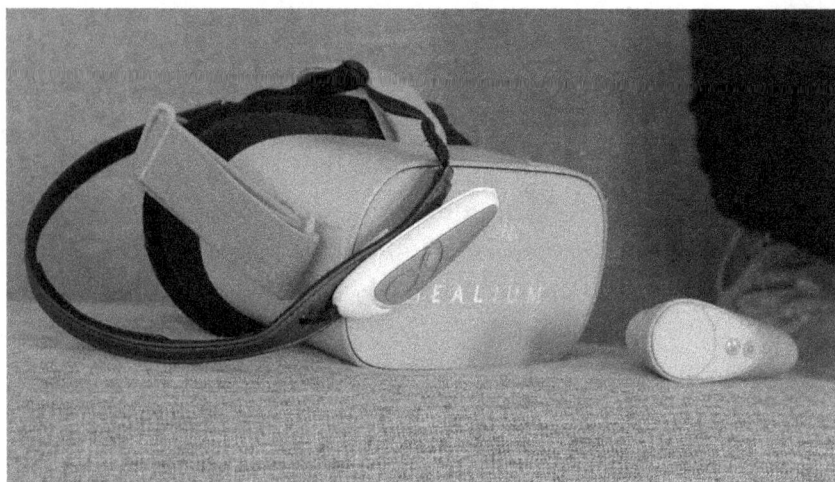

FIGURE 7.5 One example of a virtual-reality headset.

as when they become rigid and inflexible—can be related to certain concerns.

For instance, too much theta without accompanying beta often suggests a brain that is under-activated. This is a brain that may have difficulties doing its job efficiently or effectively. If this pattern shows up in the frontal lobes, the person might have difficulty inhibiting their impulses, sustaining attention, or successfully utilizing their working memory. This pattern (excessive theta/beta) is the stereotypical attention deficit hyperactivity disorder (ADHD) brainwave pattern. On the other hand, a brain that consistently has large amounts of high beta or low gamma activity, particularly when it is not needed, may show signs of anxiety, agitation, or sleep problems. This is an overactivated brain, one that is hyperaroused.

Training Your Brain with Immersive Stories

In VR, we're using two different protocols to train for specific brainwave states. Luckily, you won't need a full EEG cap to use your brainwaves with Healium as it works with consumer-grade EEG headbands. Although not diagnostic, the headband is kind of like a remote control where you're using your brain patterns to control or "heal" virtual worlds.

Quiet Mind Protocol

The Quiet Mind protocol rewards you when there is a decrease of frontal lobe activation, which occurs when you become more relaxed or reduce ruminating/worrying or excessive thinking. This protocol can be particularly helpful as an adjunctive tool if you're managing stress or reducing anxiety.

Focus Protocol

The Focus protocol rewards activation of the frontal lobes and is more useful for managing an under-aroused frontal lobe, such as what might be seen in individuals with ADHD, depression, or cognitive difficulties. The Focus protocol can be helpful for a midday mental-health break before returning to a work task or a project that needs your attention.[11]

If you're struggling with stress, anxiety, overthinking, rumination, or worry, the Quiet Mind protocol is likely to be more helpful. It is important to remember that in these scenarios you might be engaging in a brainwave pattern that may feel challenging or unknown. With this in mind, the other elements of the experience become important considerations.

Inside VR or AR, you're able to see a representation of your EEG data as a colorful aura that surrounds you. As you relax (Quiet Mind) or become more engaged and alert (Focus), the aura changes colors from yellow to green. It's almost like a traffic light controlled by your body's energy. The green color indicates success in the protocol. As long as you remain above the threshold and green, you are being successful in shifting your baseline brainwave patterns in the desired direction. You're teaching yourself to self-regulate.

When this happens, the VR experience progresses without interruption. If you happen to become stressed or unfocused during the experience, Healium's software triggers a change in the form of the aura color turning yellow. This is the feedback, helping you become more aware of your internal state.

As soon as you return to the desired state of consciousness, the aura glows green again and the experience proceeds without the "negative" yellow feedback.

VR and AR are being used in this way not only for lean back virtual relaxation but also for lean forward training. The EEG

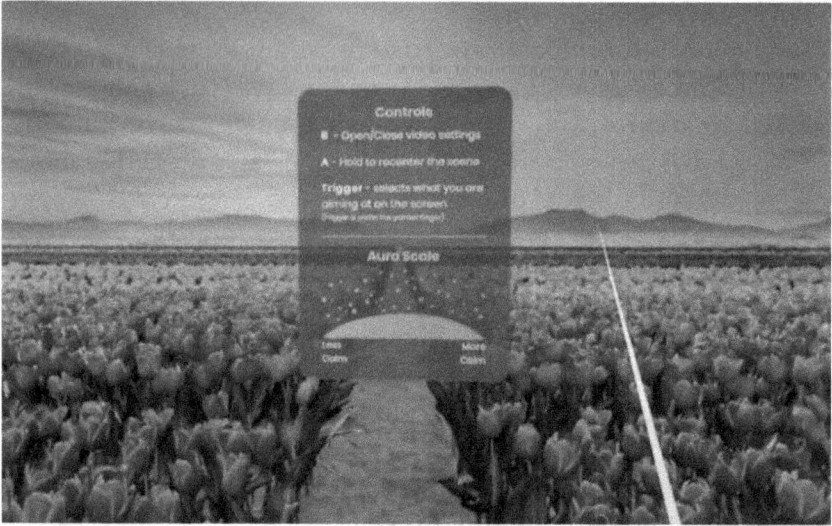

FIGURE 7.6 Inside Healium.

feedback approach is not usually recommended for acute stress reduction as it typically requires a bit of repetition to learn what internal states influence your brainwaves and the feedback. In addition, this training can take a variety of forms depending on which protocol is used, which experience is selected, how the feedback is displayed, and how the thresholds are set.

VR or AR, combined with neurofeedback, is a powerful tool to improve your media diet. Use it to improve your sleep, increase your focus, calm your mind, and rewire your thinking to reduce ruminating thoughts. More peer-reviewed research on how VR and AR impact the brain and heart is available.[12]

Remember. Your thoughts have power to control things not only in the virtual world but the real world as well.

References

1 Kropotov, J.D. (2016). Chapter 2.3: Beta and gamma rhythms. *Functional Neuromarkers for Psychiatry*, 107–119. New York: Academic Press. Retrieved from https://www.sciencedirect.com/topics/social-sciences/cultivation-theory

2 Davey, C.L.D. (2012, June 19). The psychological effects of TV news. *Psychology Today*. Retrieved from https://www.psychologytoday.com/us/blog/why-we-worry/201206/the-psychological-effects-tv-news.

3 *The Social Dilemma*. (n.d.). Retrieved from https://www.thesocialdilemma.com/

4 Neuromediation Institute. (n.d.). Retrieved from https://www.neuromeditationinstitute.com/

5 Hill, S. (2020, April 11). Your brain on stress: Understanding the stress response. *Healium*. Retrieved from https://www.tryhealium.com/2020/04/11/your-brain-on-stress-understanding-the-stress-response/

6 Healium. (n.d.). Stories: Sample our virtual and augmented reality stories. *Healium*. Retrieved from https://www.tryhealium.com/stories/

7 Tarrant, J., Vizcko, J., and Cope, H. (2018, July 24). Virtual reality for anxiety reduction demonstrated by quantitative EEG: A pilot study. *Frontiers in Psychology*. Retrieved from https://www.frontiersin.org/articles/10.3389/fpsyg.2018.01280/full

8 Tarrant, J., Abrams, J.S., and Jackson, R. (2019, September 17). The impact of virtual reality on mood states prior to blood donation. *Scholarly Journal of Psychology and Behavioral Sciences*. Retrieved from https://lupinepublishers.com/psychology-behavioral-science-journal/pdf/SJPBS.MS.ID.000150.pdf

9 Healium. (n.d.). The science behind Healium. *Healium*. Retrieved from https://www.tryhealium.com/science-behind-healium/

10 Schoengarth, B. (2020, May 22). The BrainLink Lite EEG headband: A new wearable to power Healium. *Healium*. Retrieved from https://www.tryhealium.com/2020/05/22/brainlink-lite-the-new-eeg-headband-wearable-to-power-healium/

11 Schoengarth, B. (2020, June 24). 10 moments in the day to take a mental health break. *Healium*. Retrieved from https://www.tryhealium.com/2020/06/24/10-moments-in-the-day-to-take-a-mental-health-break/

12 Healium. (n.d.). The science behind Healium. *Healium*. Retrieved from https://www.tryhealium.com/science-behind-healium/

8

Aesthetic Experiences in Healthcare

Marta Pizzolante, Marianna Graziosi,
David B. Yaden, and Alice Chirico

Imagine standing before a masterful painting, captivated by the intricate brushstrokes and vivid colors on the canvas. Or imagine a serene natural landscape, where the rustling of leaves and the sunlight through the trees transports you. These are just a couple of scenarios that illustrate aesthetic experiences. Aesthetic experiences are an important part of life involving perceiving, engaging with, and evaluating art or the inherent physical attributes of objects. They have been defined as complex and multidimensional phenomena characterized by the individual's perceptual engagement with, and cognitive appraisal of, an object, environment, or phenomenon that elicits a profound emotional response. Aesthetic experiences have been investigated by scholars across various disciplines, including philosophy, art history and psychology, as they have sought to define and understand the complex nature of aesthetic experiences. This chapter reviews scholarship and scientific work on aesthetic experiences and describes emerging virtual-reality (VR) applications in healthcare contexts.

DOI: 10.4324/9781032649771-8

Background

Psychological research has investigated the perceptive and cognitive processes behind aesthetic experiences. For example, theoretical and empirical work has examined the factors involved in why individuals tend to perceive something as "beautiful," as well as the neural mechanisms related to such perceptions. For instance, early pioneers such as Gustav Fechner studied the perceptual principles behind aesthetic experience.[1] Some behaviorists considered aesthetic experience as a kind of intrinsically motivated form of exploration, where individuals engage with art to satisfy their curiosity and intrinsic desires for novelty and complexity.[2] Contemporary advances, including the emergence of *neuroaesthetics*, employ neuroimaging methods.[3]

Although a precise and universally accepted definition of aesthetic experiences remains elusive, scholars in the fields of psychology of art and empirical aesthetics tend to converge around a shared definition. Generally, aesthetic experiences represent a unique form of subject–object relationship, in which a particular object strongly engages the subject's mind.[4] They can arise from interactions with various forms of art, nature, and everyday objects, leading to outcomes that range from pleasure, awe, and inspiration to contemplation and critical reflection. These experiences encompass three core dimensions—motivational, cognitive, and emotional processes—with related physiological, cognitive, affective, and social responses.[5] This experience is inherently subjective, varying significantly across individuals, and is influenced by a multitude of factors including cultural background, personal preferences, psychological state, and contextual circumstances. These experiences are distinguished by their ability to transcend ordinary perception, invoking a deep appreciation for beauty, form, or conceptual significance, and often result in a lasting impact on the individual's emotional well-being and cognitive processes.[6]

Beyond Beauty: Aesthetic Experiences for Human Well-being

Beyond the study of individual judgments of beauty or preference, contemporary scientific research is increasingly recognizing the well-being potential inherent in aesthetic experiences. Art and aesthetics, with their communicative nature, can evoke emotional states, and touch on profound aspects of the human condition, possessing the capability to influence well-being.[7]

Multiple perspectives and frameworks of well-being have been described. In psychology, well-being generally refers to individuals' overall life satisfaction and happiness. One prominent framework is Seligman's PERMA model, which highlights five essential elements for reaching well-being: *Positive emotion, Engagement, Relationships, Meaning, and Accomplishment* (PERMA).[8] Positive emotion refers to the presence of joy, gratitude, and contentment in one's life, emphasizing the importance of experiencing pleasurable feelings. Engagement signifies the state of flow and immersion in activities that challenge and engage one's skills and interests. Relationships are social connections and the quality of interpersonal interactions. Meaning refers to having a sense of purpose and direction in life, often derived from values, beliefs, and a sense of belonging to a larger community. Accomplishment relates to achieving goals and a sense of competence. In addition to these dimensions, well-being can be further classified into two overarching categories: hedonic and eudaimonic.[9] Hedonic well-being emphasizes the pursuit of pleasure and avoidance of pain, focusing on subjective happiness and life satisfaction. Eudaimonic well-being, on the other hand, centers on the pursuit of a meaningful and purposeful life, emphasizing personal growth, self-realization, and the actualization of one's potential.

Our focus is on the interface between aesthetic experiences and well-being, especially how aesthetic experiences can enhance it. By delving into both the hedonic and eudaimonic perspectives, we aim to add to an understanding of how aesthetic experiences can be understood in the context of enhancing well-being (see Table 8.1 for an overview of the proposed model).

Effect of aesthetic experience	Brief description	Component of PERMA Model associated	Studies referenced
Complex affective experiences	Aesthetic experiences evoke a wide range of emotions, including awe, joy, sadness, and contemplation.	P (Positive Emotions)	Konečni (2008), Schindler et al. (2017), Keltner and Haidt (2003), Shiota et al. (2007), Piff et al. (2015), Menninghaus et al. (2017), Silvia (2005, 2013), Silvia and Nusbaum (2011), Ishizu and Zeki (2011), Vessel et al. (2019), Salimpoor et al. (2015), Cross and Elizarova (2014)
Flow State	Aesthetic experiences can induce a state of deep concentration and flow, characterized by complete focus and immersion.	E (Engagement)	Csikszentmihalyi (2009, 2018), Jackson and Marsh (1996), MacDonald (2002)
Empathy and social bonding	Aesthetic experiences foster social connections, empathy, and pro-social behaviors.	R (Relationship)	Archer et al. (2015), Coulangeon and Lemel (2009), Piff et al. (2015), O'Brien (2010), Vessel et al. (2012), Rizzolatti and Craighero (2004), Molenberghs et al. (2012), Nummenmaa et al. (2008), Christov-Moore et al. (2014) Pelowski and Akiba (2011), Pelowski (2015), Lasher et al. (1983)
Epiphany and Personal Growth	Aesthetic experiences serve as a catalyst for individuals to explore and question their own existence and the broader human condition.	M (Meaning)	
Cognitive benefits: skill training	Engagement with the arts enhances cognitive skills such as analytical thinking, creativity, problem-solving, and cognitive flexibility.	A (Accomplishments)	Hennessey and Amabile (1987), Leder et al. (2004, 2016), Cupchik and Winston (1996), Bolwerk et al. (2014), Winner and Hetland (2000), Chan et al. (2017), Hanna-Pladdy and Mackay (2011), Pinho et al. (2014)

TABLE 8.1 Aesthetic experience effects, explanation and associated component of the PERMA model
Note: See Endnotes for complete citations.

In the following subsections, we address each dimension described by the PERMA model.

Positive Emotions: The Emotional Impact of Aesthetic Experiences

Aesthetic experiences elicit emotions. It is well known that the arts have the power to resonate with individuals on an emotional level, creating a feeling of connection between the artwork, the artist, and the observer.[10]

Although these emotions, which have been termed "aesthetic," encompass a wide range of perceptions, they all share the same common thread of appreciating and assessing beauty, meaning, or significance.[11] Aesthetic experiences are about evaluating and appreciating objects or events in an aesthetic context, and art, nature, or other stimuli can trigger these emotions.[12] Specifically, what unites these diverse experiences is the inherent aesthetic appraisal intertwined with the emotional response. In other words, aesthetic emotions are not only about emotional impact but also about evaluating the aesthetic qualities inherent in the stimulus. For instance, awe induced by art and aesthetics—which can be assimilated to the sublime[13]—is characterized by experiencing conflicting emotions, induced by the perception of vastness in which individuals are confronted with something greater than themselves, leading to a need to accommodate this profound experience.[14] Due to this emotional depth, the experience becomes more enriched, providing individuals with the opportunity to delve into emotional subtleties and ambiguities, a phenomenon often ignited by art that leads to profound introspection and personal growth.[15] A range of positive outcomes have been found to be associated with experiencing awe through art, including epistemic expansion—the process of expanding knowledge, understanding, and awareness of various concepts, ideas, or domains of knowledge—increased pro-social behavior, as well as a broader perspective on life.[16]

There are individual differences related to aesthetic experience and their emotional responses. Researchers have found that personal factors, such as personality traits, cultural background, and past experiences, affect how people interpret and respond to art emotionally.[17] A high level of openness to experience, for example, may be more open to novel and unconventional forms of art, whereas a preference for structure and order may be attracted to traditional and representational forms of art.[18]

Several brain regions are involved in aesthetic experiences, including the prefrontal cortex, the insula, the anterior cingulate cortex, and the limbic system.[19] They play a role in emotional processing, memory retrieval, and reward processing. In response to art that elicits emotions, such as joy or awe, these brain regions are activated, leading to a cascade of neural responses that contribute to the overall emotional experience.[20]

Neuroimaging techniques, such as functional magnetic resonance imaging (fMRI), have provided insights into aesthetic emotions. Vessel et al. examined the brain responses to different art genres and found that each genre produced unique patterns of brain activity.[21] Abstract art activated brain regions associated with self-referential processing and introspection. Comparatively, representational art engages brain regions related to object recognition and contextual processing. These findings suggest that art engages distinct cognitive processes as well as elicits emotions.

Music also generates aesthetic emotions. Music has been demonstrated to elicit awe, depending upon individuals' musical preferences and personality traits, i.e., need for cognition and cognitive closure.[22] Music can, of course, evoke other intense emotions, such as joy, sadness, or nostalgia.[23] The amygdala and orbitofrontal cortex exhibit increased activity when individuals listen to emotionally charged music.[24]

Performing arts, such as theater and dance, can also promote a huge variety of aesthetic emotional states. Observers of dance can resonate with the emotional states portrayed by the dancers when dance evokes emotional contagion.[25] In dance, visual and kinesthetic elements combine to evoke a shared emotional experience, demonstrating the capacity of nonverbal communication and evocation.

Engagement: Art and the Flow State

Engagement, as outlined in the PERMA model, signifies a state of complete absorption and immersion in an activity or experience, often accompanied by a sense of timelessness and heightened focus.[26] Research indicates that aesthetic engagement can induce a heightened state of flow, described as an optimal psychological condition where individuals become wholly absorbed in a task or activity.[27] This flow state is characterized by a match between the individual's skills and the challenges posed by the activity, resulting in a sense of complete focus and immersion.[28] Within this state, individuals often experience reduced self-consciousness. Time also takes on a unique quality in the flow state, with individuals perceiving its passage differently—sometimes quickly, other times slowing down. This altered sense of time enhances the immersive and fulfilling nature of the flow state, making it a remarkable psychological condition where individuals become wholly absorbed in their task or activity, leading to heightened engagement, creativity, and overall well-being.[29]

The concept of flow has connections to aesthetic engagement.[30] Early studies conducted on the theme have demonstrated that activities such as artistic creation, musical expression, or writing can lead individuals to experience flow, where time seems to pass effortlessly, and a profound sense of fulfillment is achieved. Flow has been linked to enhanced creativity[31] and possibly improved performance,[32] as well as increased well-being.[33] Importantly, this state is not exclusive to accomplished artists; both artists and laypeople can immerse themselves in captivating artistic activities and achieve the flow state. For instance, a study by MacDonald explored the experiences of laypeople participating in various artistic endeavors, such as drawing, singing, and dancing. Participants reported feelings of intense focus, enjoyment, and a sense of losing track of time during these activities, indicative of a flow state.[34]

Relationship: Fostering Empathy and Social Bonding through Aesthetic Experience

Aesthetic experiences may foster social connections and pro-social behaviors in some cases.[35] For example, awe experiences have been demonstrated to be elicited among close relationships.[36] Furthermore, aesthetic encounters have been shown to be related to empathy disposition and compassion.[37]

The arts can foster social connection.[38] Attending cultural events or engaging in shared aesthetic activities creates communal experiences, strengthening social bonds and fostering a sense of belonging.[39] As an example, Coulangeon and Lemel found that individuals engaging in cultural activities, such as art exhibitions, theater performances, or music concerts, reported a higher sense of social integration, fostering a sense of community.[40] Milne and Otieno investigated the effects of art education on empathy among school children, revealing that students participating in art programs exhibited improved empathy.[41] Additionally, research has demonstrated that awe-inspiring experiences, often triggered by encounters with art or natural beauty, were linked to increased altruistic behavior.[42] Lastly, O'Brien established a relationship between cultural engagement and community well-being, showing that communities with higher levels of cultural participation tended to exhibit greater social cohesion and overall well-being.[43]

Regarding neural underpinnings associated with this mechanism, Vessel and colleagues found that when participants viewed aesthetically pleasing images, they exhibited greater activation in brain areas associated with empathy and emotion regulation.[44] These cohesive effects of the arts can be attributed to several interrelated neural mechanisms rooted in the functioning of the human social brain. One of these mechanisms is the concept of mirror neurons, which has been extensively explored within the artistic domain.[45] Mirror neurons are specialized neurons in the brain that fire both when an individual performs an action and when they observe another person performing the same action.[46] Through this discovery, neuroscientific research found out the ways in which we empathize with others, highlighting the role of implicit patterns of others' behaviors and experiences. Additionally, mirror neurons may contribute to the phenomenon of emotional contagion in social settings.[47] However, the specific role of mirror neurons in such cases is still being explored and should be considered exploratory.

Other neural mechanisms associated with classical conditioning and associative learning, as well as neuroendocrine mechanisms involving oxytocin and prolactin, may play vital roles in mediating the reward and emotional responses triggered by aesthetic encounters.[48] Moreover, the social touch mechanisms, linked to the activation of cutaneous mechanoreceptors, may contribute to the emotional bonding that arises during shared aesthetic experiences.

Meaning: Art for Epiphany and Personal Growth

Meaning is the sense of purpose and significance individuals find in their lives, encompassing the belief that their actions and existence matter in a broader context.[49] Art frequently serves as a catalyst for individuals to explore and question their own existence and the broader human condition. These encounters have the potential to unveil hidden truths, challenge established norms, and inspire fresh perspectives. This potential has been progressively recognized by the scientific literature as "transformative." In a recent conceptual analysis, Chirico and colleagues defined transformative experiences as "brief experiences, perceived as extraordinary and unique, entailing durable and/or irreversible outcomes, which contribute to changing individuals' self-conception, worldviews, and view of others, as well as their own personality and identity."[50] The authors identified two pivotal components that underpin transformative experiences: epistemic expansion and emotional complexity. In addition to these phenomenological elements, two psychological elements were determined as relevant for the scope of the systematic review: facilitating conditions or elicitors, and specific effects on the recipient, often referred to as aftereffects.

In line with this, Pelowski and Akiba emphasized the need to move beyond mere cognitive mastery and perceptual pleasure in understanding aesthetic experiences.[51] They argued that focusing solely on these aspects can limit the experience from a viewer's personal beliefs and identity, limiting the potential for art to deeply impact lives. They highlighted the importance of addressing discrepant experiences during an art encounter, particularly when a beholder's expectations are violated, leading to a metacognitive reassessment of the artwork and eventual self-schema transformation. Similarly, several authors emphasized the role of the arts in mental and emotional growth, highlighting their capacity to engage individuals in representational conflicts that, when resolved, facilitate the restructuring and unification of initial mental representations.[52]

Pelowski et al. proposed an empirical approach to study art experiences in the context of self-transformation and understanding.[53] For instance, the Vienna Integrated Model of Art Perception (VIMAP) combines bottom-up and top-down processes to better understand how individuals perceive and interact with visual art, revealing emotional, evaluative, and physiological factors.[54] As an example, the act of feeling like (or actually) crying during an art experience, which is coupled with specific emotional and cognitive responses, can serve as a physical indicator of transformation, to the self-reflection, shifted perspectives, and self-schema changes.[55]

Accomplishments: Art's Cognitive Perks

Accomplishments encapsulate the sense of achievement and personal growth that individuals experience when they pursue and attain meaningful goals.[56] In the context of art and aesthetic experiences, accomplishments can be seen as one of the tangible outcomes resulting from creative endeavors. These achievements can range from mastering a musical instrument to completing a challenging painting, writing a novel, or successfully choreographing a dance performance. The process of setting artistic goals, working to achieve them, and ultimately realizing one's creative vision contributes to a profound sense of accomplishment and personal fulfillment.

Visual arts, music, and performing arts often demand innovative thinking, encouraging individuals to explore new perspectives and experiment with unconventional solutions.[57] As Leder and colleagues point out, when individuals immerse themselves in visual artworks, they embark on a cognitive journey of deciphering symbols, metaphors, and visual narratives.[58] This decoding process requires the viewer to analyze and synthesize information, make connections between visual elements, and extract meaning from the composition. Such mental activities stimulate analytical thinking, encouraging individuals to explore various perspectives and engage in critical reflection.

Furthermore, research by Cupchik and Winston highlights how the ambiguity and open-ended nature of many artworks encourage viewers to generate multiple interpretations and solutions.[59] This cognitive flexibility not only enhances analytical thinking but also nurtures creativity and the ability to consider alternative perspectives—a valuable skill in problem solving across various domains. Conversely, the process of creating art not only fosters perceptual and motor skills but also engages higher-order cognitive functions. Artistic creation entails meticulous planning, decision making, and critical thinking, all of which contribute to the refinement of executive functions.[60] Research conducted by Winner and Hetland underscores the role of arts education in nurturing divergent thinking, a cognitive skill relevant for generating creative ideas.[61] This capacity to navigate a huge variety of mental pathways not only promote artistic expression but also translates to other cognitive domains, yielding advantages in problem-solving and innovation. In another study by Chan and colleagues, participants who actively partook in art classes (specifically Chinese calligraphy writing) demonstrated notable enhancements in attention, working memory, and problem-solving skills.[62]

Aesthetic appreciation of music extends its cognitive reach to auditory processing and cognitive flexibility. The complexity of musical structures, along with the need to synchronize rhythm and melody, sharpens auditory discrimination and temporal processing skills.[63] Additionally, musical improvisation fosters cognitive flexibility and divergent thinking by encouraging individuals to spontaneously generate novel melodies and harmonies.[64]

The Decalogue for Integrating Aesthetic Experiences and New Tech in Healthcare

1. *User-Centered Design:* Start by placing the patient at the center of the design process. Consider their preferences, needs, and comfort levels when creating VR or art-based experiences. Ensure that the technology is accessible to a wide range of individuals, including those with physical or cognitive limitations.

2. *Emotionally Engaging Content:* Develop content that elicits positive emotions, such as joy, relaxation, and inspiration. Aesthetic experiences should aim to uplift the patient's mood and reduce stress. This can involve soothing visuals, calming audio, or immersive storytelling.

3. *Personalization:* Tailor the experiences to the individual patient's preferences and therapeutic goals. Some patients may find solace in serene natural landscapes, while others might prefer more abstract or artistic visuals. Offering choices and customization can enhance the effectiveness of the intervention.

4. *Therapeutic Integration:* Collaborate closely with healthcare professionals, psychologists, and therapists to ensure that the aesthetic experiences align with therapeutic objectives. Integrate these

experiences into existing treatment plans and strategies for managing specific medical conditions.

5. *Measurement and Assessment:* Implement ways to measure the impact of the aesthetic experiences on patient well-being. Collect data on emotional responses, stress levels, and patient-reported outcomes to continuously improve the effectiveness of the interventions.

6. *Ethical Considerations:* Address ethical concerns surrounding patient privacy, consent, and the potential for overstimulation in VR environments. Ensure that patients are well-informed about the technology and its purpose, and respect their autonomy in choosing to participate.

7. *Accessibility and Inclusivity:* Make sure that the technology and experiences are accessible to all patients, including those with disabilities. Consider features like adjustable font sizes, voice commands, or alternative input methods for patients who may have physical limitations.

8. *Training and Support:* Provide adequate training and support to both healthcare staff and patients to maximize the benefits of the technology. Educate healthcare providers on how to incorporate these experiences into patient care effectively.

9. *Research and Iteration:* Continuously evaluate and iterate on the aesthetic experiences based on scientific research and patient feedback. As the field evolves, update the guidelines and practices accordingly to stay at the forefront of healthcare technology.

10. *Collaboration and Partnerships:* Foster collaborations between healthcare institutions, technology developers, artists, and researchers. Cross-disciplinary partnerships can lead to innovative solutions and a deeper understanding of the therapeutic potential of new technologies in healthcare.

Aesthetic Experiences in Healthcare

In the realm of healthcare, the potential of art, music, and other aesthetic experiences has garnered significant attention in recent years. Beyond their general impact on well-being, these creative modalities have shown some evidence for their impact on the health and recovery of patients in clinical settings.

There is evidence for the growing recognition of the value of the arts in improving well-being, health, and healthcare worldwide. According to recent reports by the World Health Organization (WHO), more than 80% of the world's countries now acknowledge the therapeutic benefits of incorporating arts and creativity into healthcare settings.[65] In the United States alone, the National Endowment for the Arts (NEA) reported that over 3,000 healthcare organizations have implemented art-based programs, serving approximately 3 million patients annually.[66] Moreover, several research published by the *British Journal of Psychiatry* indicated that art-therapy programs in Europe have increased by nearly 40% in the past decade.[67] These statistics underscore the global recognition of the positive impact that art, music, and other aesthetic experiences can have on promoting well-being and fostering healing in healthcare environments.

Art-based practices in healthcare offer numerous potential benefits. Firstly, these practices provide a noninvasive and nonpharmacological approach to healing, making them accessible to diverse patient populations. Secondly, art-based interventions tap into the creative potential of individuals, fostering self-expression, empowerment, emotional processing, and the cognitive "perks" outlined above. Thirdly, these practices may promote holistic healing by engaging the mind, body, and emotions, addressing the interconnected aspects of well-being. Lastly, art-based practices offer a versatile and adaptable therapeutic tool, applicable in various healthcare settings, from mental-health facilities to palliative care, supporting patients' transformative journeys toward improved well-being and quality of life across the lifespan.

Art therapy is grounded in the belief that art possesses therapeutic potential, impacting both physical and mental well-being.

This approach is involves using art-based interventions to address various medical conditions.[68] These interventions encompass experiencing art, such as viewing paintings or listening to music, and creating art, like painting or dancing. The underlying premise is that engaging with art triggers physiological and mental processes, influencing body and brain systems relevant to somatic and psychological health.

In the following sections, various practices, and domains of use of aesthetic experiences in the healthcare context are explored (see Table 8.2 for an overview).

Art Therapy: Nurturing Emotional Expression and Communication in Mental Health and Chronic Illness

Art therapy is a well-established practice in the domain of art-based healthcare. It involves the use of various artistic mediums, such as painting, drawing, and sculpting, to facilitate emotional expression and communication.[69] Particularly salient for individuals navigating trauma, chronic illnesses, or other mental-health challenges, art therapy offers a profound outlet for those who may struggle to convey their emotions through traditional verbal means. In the therapeutic process, patients are encouraged to engage in creative activities, inviting them to externalize intricate emotions and delve into their inner worlds.[70] Through this process, patients often gain profound insights into their emotional dynamics, by promoting self-awareness and personal development. The creative act itself may become a cathartic release, enabling individuals to confront and process challenging experiences within a safe and supportive environment.

Empirical evidence shows evidence for a possible impact of art therapy on psychological well-being. Engaging with art has been shown to lead to modest reductions in anxiety, depression, and stress levels among patients.[71] In a scoping review, Fancourt and Finn examined all the studies on the transformative potential of art therapy, revealing how art-therapy interventions were associated with positive psychological changes and post-traumatic growth among individuals grappling with acquired brain injuries.[72]

In a randomized controlled trial with cancer patients, Monti and colleagues demonstrated the profound effects of mindfulness-based art therapy (MBAT), where a significant decrease in stress levels after participation in art-therapy sessions for patients who engaged in art therapy when compared with a wait-list control group.[73] Furthermore, a recent meta-analysis looking across 14 studies at MBAT, researchers found evidence for a medium-sized effect of the efficacy of these interventions in reducing symptoms of depression, anxiety, and fatigue.[74]

Music Therapy: Easing Stress and Anxiety for Patients and Caregivers in Hospitals

Music therapy uses sound and rhythm to enhance the emotional well-being and general health of patients, from pediatric patients undergoing medical procedures to elderly residents in long-term care facilities, again underscoring the potential of aesthetic experiences across the lifespan.[75] This therapeutic approach encompasses various music-based interventions, including activities like listening to music, engaging in singing, or playing musical instruments, all tailored to address a diverse spectrum of physical, emotional, and cognitive needs.[76]

Empirical investigations have provided some evidence that music therapy may help alleviate pain, stress, and anxiety levels in patients enduring medical procedures or grappling with persistent conditions. Research has found some evidence for this potential in patients with cancer[77] and depression.[78] Furthermore, this type of therapy may help with coping mechanisms and resilience, consequently contributing to more favorable overall treatment outcomes.[79] Within healthcare domains, music therapy functions as a tool for pain management and cultivating a soothing ambiance, thereby ameliorating emotional distress, and fostering relaxation. A systematic review of 42 randomized controlled trials (RCTs) found that music interventions had positive effects on reducing anxiety and pain in roughly half of the studies included.[80] For example, a RCT conducted by Nilsson and colleagues examined postoperative pain among patients recovering from abdominal surgery.[81] The study's cohort of 75 participants was divided into two groups: one receiving standard care and the other receiving both standard care and music therapy sessions. Outcomes revealed that the music therapy recipients reported diminished pain intensity and reduced reliance on pain medication in comparison to the control group. In the realm of dementia, music therapy exhibits promise in elevating the quality of life for affected individuals. For instance, Guetin and colleagues explored the effects of music therapy on behavioral and psychological symptoms of dementia (BPSD).[82] Their RCT with 60 participants underlined the efficacy of music therapy interventions in significantly mitigating agitation and anxiety among individuals with dementia. Silverman conducted a randomized study over the course of a 12-week group music therapy intervention for individuals with schizophrenia, finding marked enhancements in social functioning and overall emotional well-being in the music therapy group.[83] Music therapy has also found application within neurological rehabilitation settings. A systematic review of 23 studies examining the effects of rhythmic auditory stimulation (RAS)—a music-based intervention involving rhythmic cues—on motor function in stroke patients found that this modality was associated with significant improvement in arm motor function.[84]

Nature-Based Interventions: Cultivating Resilience and Posttraumatic Growth Amid the Healing Process

Nature-based interventions, also known as ecotherapy, have been studied extensively in various healthcare settings, demonstrating some potential in promoting well-being and healing among individuals with different conditions.[85] These experiences, often involving activities in natural settings such as gardening, forest bathing (i.e., spending time in forest nature environments), or simply spending time in green spaces, can be considered aesthetic experiences.

One study found that patients recovering from surgery who had views of nature from their hospital rooms experienced lower stress levels and required less pain medication compared to those with views of a brick wall.[86] Several more recent studies have found that the presence of foliage in hospital rooms of patients recovering from surgery had positive and therapeutic effects on patient mood and recovery.[87] Nature walks have also been associated with improved mental-health outcomes including reduced rumination, a common symptom of depression and anxiety, promoting a more positive mood and cognitive functioning.[88] Nature-based interventions, such as forest bathing or spending time in natural settings, have been associated with reduced cortisol levels, a hormone linked to stress.[89] These findings highlight the possible stress-reducing effects of nature-based therapies, making them valuable tools in managing stress-related disorders like anxiety and depression.

Interacting with nature has been shown to improve cognitive functioning and attention restoration. A review by Hartig and colleagues emphasized that spending time in natural environments, particularly urban green spaces, can enhance attention and working memory as indicated by their review of the literature.[90] Nature walks have been associated with improved scores on cognitive tests related to attention and memory.[91] A systematic review of observational studies by Annerstedt and Währborg indicated that nature-based interventions improved cognitive function and increased overall well-being among individuals with dementia.[92]

Even exposure to nature in VR was found to promote parasympathetic nervous system activity and facilitate recovery from tress among healthy participants.[93] Nature-based therapies offer a promising approach for cognitive rehabilitation.

Nature-based interventions have been used in trauma recovery programs to support emotional healing and post-traumatic growth. This intersection of aesthetic experience and healthcare has been most widely studied among veterans, though empirical work is still needed.[94] In a systematic review by Poulson and colleagues, the authors concluded that nature-based therapies were associated with improved ability of veterans to deal with posttraumatic stress disorder (PTSD) symptoms as well as lowered stress and improved well-being.[95] In a more recent study by Anderson and colleagues, the level of awe experienced by military veterans engaging in nature-based therapy predicted these participants' increased well-being scores and decreased stress responses at a one-week follow-up.[96] This suggests that the aesthetic experience of engaging with the natural environment, which may evoke feelings of awe and wonder, is a mechanism of change that warrants further investigation.

Dance and Movement Therapy: Integrating Mind and Body for Rehabilitation and Mental Health

Dance and movement therapies leverage the connection between the mind and body to promote holistic healing and emotional expression.[97] This therapeutic approach involves using guided movement and dance techniques to facilitate emotional exploration and integration, bridging the gap between the conscious and unconscious aspects of oneself.[98]

Dance and movement therapy has shown promising results in the treatment of individuals with eating disorders. A study by Savidaki and colleagues examined the effects of dance movement

Art-based therapy type	Targeted condition	Studies referenced
Visual art therapy	Trauma, chronic illnesses, mental-health challenges	Malchiodi (2012), Stuckey and Nobel (2010), Finn and Fancourt (2018), van Lith et al. (2018), Monti et al. (2006)
Music therapy	Stress, anxiety, pain management, dementia, mental-health conditions, neurological rehabilitation	Gold et al. (2009), Gold and Mahrer (2018), Bradt et al. (2015, 2016), Chan et al. (2003), Raglio et al. (2016), Nilsson et al. (2005), Guetin et al. (2009), Silverman (2019)
Nature-based interventions	Stress, anxiety, depression, cognitive functioning, dementia, trauma recovery	Bratman et al. (2015), Ulrich (1984), Berman et al. (2012), Hartig et al. (2014), Annerstedt et al. (2013)
Dance and movement therapy	Eating disorders, palliative care, trauma recovery	Meekums (2002), Payne et al. (2016), Bradt et al. (2015)

TABLE 8.2 Art-based therapy, healthcare targets, and relevant literature
Notes: See Endnotes for complete citations.

therapy on body image and self-esteem among individuals with anorexia nervosa.[99] The findings revealed that dance movement therapy interventions led to modest improvements in body image perception and increased self-esteem. Engaging in expressive and creative movement allows individuals to reconnect with their bodies in a positive and nonjudgmental way, fostering a more accepting and compassionate relationship with oneself.[100]

In palliative-care settings, dance and movement therapy provides a means of self-expression, dignity, and connection during end-of-life experiences.[101] The embodied nature of dance and movement allows patients to communicate and process their emotions nonverbally, especially when verbal communication becomes challenging or insufficient. Studies have shown that dance and movement therapy interventions in palliative-care settings promote emotional well-being and improve patients' quality of life.[102] The creative and expressive nature of dance can allow some patients to foster a sense of agency in the face of illness.[103]

Dance therapy has also been used in trauma recovery programs to support emotional healing and posttraumatic growth. Research by Burns explored the use of dance movement therapy in survivors of sexual assault.[104] The findings revealed that dance movement therapy provided a safe space for individuals to process their trauma, expressing emotions and experiences through movement. The embodied nature of dance can help some individuals access emotions stored in the body, promoting emotional release and resilience.[105] Dance and movement therapy can be particularly helpful for individuals who struggle with verbal expression, providing an alternative and embodied mode of communication and healing.

Innovative Applications: Aesthetic Experiences and New Immersive Technology for Human Health

In recent years, the interest in the scientific understanding of well-being, together with the rapid advancement of technology, has opened up a new realm of possible psychological applications.[106] Specifically, Immersive Technologies (i.e., virtual, augmented, or mixed reality) have garnered increasing attention for their potential applications in healthcare. VR immerses users in a fully digital environment, shutting out the physical world and replacing it with a computer-generated one. Augmented reality (AR) enhances the real world by overlaying digital information or objects onto our physical surroundings. Mixed reality (MR) combines elements of both VR and AR, allowing digital and physical objects to interact in real time. VR is among the most promising of these in the near term.

These technologies have the unique ability to immerse users into realistic virtual worlds, generating a profound sense of presence, immersion, and engagement, fostering positive change.[107] Additionally, the combination of immersive technology and aesthetics potentially represents a new frontier for human well-being enhancement.

In the following sections, we delve into the multifaceted role of a particular immersive technology, especially VR, within healthcare settings. We also explore how VR, in its pioneering integration with art and aesthetic experiences, can contribute to transformative applications in the realm of healthcare.

Immersive Technologies for Enhanced Well-Being and Positive Change: The Potential of Virtual Reality

The field of positive technology, at the intersection of psychology and technology, studies information, and communication technology (ICT) and its impacts on individuals, groups, and institutions, with a primary focus on well-being. Drawing inspiration from influential past research, this field studies the potential of technology to enhance well-being.[108]

VR stands out for its unique capacity to immerse users in customized environments, crafting experiences that not only replicate physical settings but also offer opportunities for enhancing overall well-being and emotional resilience.[109] VR involves several factors that make it a compelling technology: immersion, which refers to its capacity to draw individuals into the virtual world; presence, making the virtual environment feel tangible and real; and engagement, capturing users' attention and evoking emotional involvement. These dimensions are better defined in subsequent sections in the attempt to integrate art and aesthetic experiences in the virtual realm.

Through the replication of sensory inputs (such as visual and auditory stimuli) and motor interactions (including immersive settings and motion tracking) akin to those encountered in the physical world, VR has the capability to construct a subjective encounter that is a convincing simulation of reality.[110] VR is frequently described as an "advanced imaginal system," because it represents an experiential form of mental imagery renowned for its effectiveness in evoking emotional responses.[111]

Many of the studies explored the potential of VR for patients struggling with mental-health concerns. Research has been conducted on eating disorders[112] and mood disorders such as depression and anxiety.[113] VR-based treatments for exposure therapies may be suitable for patients to confront fears in a controlled setting, resulting in symptom reduction.[114] In the domain of cognitive and motor-skill enhancement, several studies on VR-based stroke rehabilitation linked heightened presence with improved motor function and daily outcomes.[115]

Recent research has examined the potential of VR for promoting well-being. For example, Enrique and colleagues tested an adaptation which integrated a "Best Possible Self" exercise, which encourages positive future-oriented thinking, integrated within a self-guided VR platform.[116] The authors found that this adaptation was able to improve future expectations and reduce depressive symptoms for a brief period, though these changes were not maintained at three-month follow-up.

VR's immersive qualities also aid chronic pain management by diverting attention from pain stimuli.[117] VR-based relaxation techniques complement this approach, reducing stress and anxiety levels for holistic pain management. In the realm of mental health, VR holds promise for treating PTSD, as indicated in a study by Rothbaum and colleagues that exposed individuals with PTSD to virtual recreations of traumatic events, resulting in significant symptom reduction.[118]

In pediatric healthcare, VR is leveraged for distraction and pain management during medical procedures, with several studies conducted by Gold and colleagues demonstrating reduced pain and distress levels in children who experience VR.[119]

Emotion regulation is a crucial aspect of well-being, and it has been extensively studied also in the context of integrating various technologies, including VR.[120] An increasing number of authors is suggesting VR as the ultimate "empathy machine," employed to specifically promote empathy, altruism, and a deeper understanding of others.[121]

VR has been particularly promising in the study of awe.[122] Notably, Stepanova and colleagues provided a comprehensive framework for designing virtual experiences that induce the "overview effect,"[123] which refers to the of awe and self-transcendence that astronauts report experiencing when gazing at the earth from space.[124] This experience aims to cultivate feelings of awe, interconnectedness, and environmental responsibility among users.

By exploring these various aspects, VR technology demonstrates its potential to positively impact well-being, which may have some useful implications for healthcare settings.

Exploring New Horizons: Art and Aesthetics in Virtual Environments

The convergence of art, aesthetics, and immersive technology is opening new avenues for creative expression. VR is a new artistic medium that artists are exploring. Digital artists like Refik Anadol (https://acuteart.com/marina-abramovic-first-virtual-reality-artwork-to-be-presented-at-the-58th-venice-biennale/; https://www.zacharyrichter.com/life-of-us) in pieces like "Melting Memories" and others, Anadol translated brain-activity data into an immersive visual experience. In another example, "Infinity Room" creates the sensation of a space without limits.[125] Additionally, artists like Marina Abramović have explored VR's emotional depth. Her project "Rising" immersed viewers in the effects of climate change. Chris Milk's "Life of Us" allows users to evolve through time, exemplifying VR's potential for collaborative storytelling.

Traditional barriers separating observers from artworks can seem to dissolve at times when individuals step into virtual realms, becoming co-creator of the aesthetic experience itself.[126] That is, not only VR can accurately evoke the same emotional responses as real-life art,[127] but it is able to promote an even stronger emotional experience, often of a multisensory nature, where viewers are completely immersed within the artist's creation or the aesthetic stimuli.[128]

This is possible thanks to the simultaneous presence of three fundamental dimensions in VR: immersion, sense of presence, and engagement. According to Slater and Wilbur, immersion refers to the extent to which individuals feel completely absorbed in the virtual environment, relying on the objective technological capabilities of the device to provide a varied array of multisensory stimulation, and tracking that maintain fidelity to real-world sensory modalities.[129] The immersive nature of VR provides users an environment where they can interact with and manipulate artworks in ways not possible through traditional mediums.[130]

The sense of presence pertains to the feeling of "being there" within the virtual environment, as if it were a genuine, tangible space. VR technologies are adept at creating a convincing illusion of presence, allowing individuals to forget, at least temporarily, the physical world around them.[131]

Engagement encompasses the level of active participation and involvement of individuals within the virtual environment. VR offers a dynamic and interactive platform where viewers can actively engage with artworks, manipulate elements, and navigate the virtual space at their own pace. This interactivity promotes a sense of agency and ownership over the aesthetic experience, transforming individuals from passive spectators into active participants in the creation and exploration of art.

In this regard, VR has shown efficacy in eliciting emotionally resonant experiences—intense emotional responses, closely mirroring or intensifying the feelings typically associated with real-world stimuli or events.

Researchers are increasingly testing this, exploring how VR-mediated artistic experiences influence emotional responses, cognitive engagement, and physiological markers.[132]

Crafting Transformative Experiences: Architecting Aesthetic Journeys through Immersive Technologies in Healthcare

Aesthetic experiences brought about by new technologies may have some potential applications in healthcare settings. In recent years, the inclusion of art-based practices with healthcare has led to using new technologies to promote well-being and enhance therapeutic outcomes. The incorporation of aesthetically pleasing elements into healthcare environments has shown promising results. There is a growing body of evidence indicating that enhancing the patient experience through these elements can lead to higher levels of patient satisfaction and improved recovery rates.[133]

With the rise of telehealth therapy, it becomes increasingly apparent that tools like VR have immense potential in assisting patients with sensory, cognitive, and motor-related disabilities.[134] These individuals often face obstacles when trying to engage with traditional art media in therapeutic contexts, making alternative creative outlets a necessity and a powerful means by which to reduce barriers to access such treatments.[135]

Art-based practices have long been recognized for their therapeutic benefits, and when coupled with immersive technologies like VR, they become even more potent tools for healing and personal growth. However, despite these evident advantages, the implementation of VR and art-based practices in healthcare settings remains limited. However, despite the clear advantages they offer, the widespread integration of VR and art-based therapies in healthcare settings remains limited, prompting the need for a comprehensive examination of the underlying factors hindering their adoption.

One of the primary challenges contributing to this limited adoption is the issue of technological accessibility. High-quality VR equipment can be costly, necessitating significant financial investments for healthcare institutions.[136] Moreover, specialized training is often required for both healthcare professionals and patients to effectively utilize these technologies.[137]

Another critical consideration pertains to regulatory and ethical concerns surrounding the use of VR in healthcare. The integration of VR technologies raises complex issues related to patient consent, data privacy, and medical ethics.[138]

Furthermore, while the potential therapeutic benefits of VR and art-based practices are promising, the lack of robust empirical studies and clinical trials often hinders their evidence-based implementation in healthcare contexts.[139]

Effective integration of VR and art-based therapies also necessitates interdisciplinary collaboration among experts in fields such as art therapy, psychology, medicine, and technology.[140] Achieving seamless cooperation and communication among these diverse disciplines is crucial for the development of comprehensive and patient-centric interventions.

In conclusion, the integration of VR and art-based therapeutic practices holds significant promise for enhancing healing and personal growth within healthcare settings. However, addressing the multifaceted challenges of technological accessibility is imperative to fully unlock the potential of these innovative approaches in the realm of healthcare.

Conclusions

In this review, our aim is to describe the relationship between aesthetic experiences and well-being. These experiences encompass a wide spectrum, ranging from the nuanced details in visual art, vast and immersive natural landscapes, and the evocative harmonies of music. Within the realm of healthcare, art-based practices are increasingly common, and new immersive technologies are providing new potential interventions.

However, the potential of aesthetic experience interventions must be accompanied with caution. For example, intense emotions can lead to emotional distress and discomfort, necessitating careful handling by trained professionals.[141] Additionally, caution is needed when eliciting positive emotions in participants with a history of bipolar I disorder.[142] When integrating any aesthetic intervention into the healthcare settings, the same degree of scrutiny must be exercised as in any kind of intervention.

There are ethical considerations in this domain as well. It is essential to obtain fully informed consent from patients. Of particular importance here is to ensure that patients are informed of what aesthetic interventions may be able to offer them, as well as the limitations of these interventions on prognosis of our outcome of a given medical presentation. The cultural sensitivity of artistic content adds another layer of complexity, as certain images, symbols, or themes might carry culturally specific connotations that could be inappropriate, distressing, and/or offensive for certain individuals. Furthermore, as aesthetic interventions become more integrated into healthcare, a code of ethics may be developed; however, until such a code exists, practitioners must default to the code of ethics associated with their credential and consider the impact of aesthetic interventions in the context of such a code.[143]

We have described research on some of the well-being benefits of aesthetic experiences, such as awe and others. While this research is promising, it should be considered largely preliminary as replications are needed. Also, effect sizes are generally modest. New immersive technologies such as VR are particularly promising in this domain, due to the feelings of presence and interactive aspects it affords. We discussed some potential applications of aesthetic experiences for the purpose of well-being delivered through VR technologies in healthcare settings as well as cautions. We believe that it is worth considering how to capture some of life's most interesting experiences and convey them to those who could benefit from them most, such as those in healthcare settings.

References

1 Gepshtein, S. (2010). Two psychologies of perception and the prospect of their synthesis. *Philosophical Psychology*, *23*(2), 217–281.

2 See, for example, Barnes, M.E. (2009). Behaviorism and aesthetics? The life and career of Daniel E. Berlyne. Library and Archives Canada, Bibliothèque et Archives Canada, Ottawa.

3 Zeki, S., Bao, Y., & Pöppel, E. (2020). Neuroaesthetics: The art, science, and brain triptych. *PsyCh Journal*, *9*(4), 427–428.

4 Ognjenović, P. (1997). *Psihološka teorija umetnosti* [*Psychological theory of art*]. Belgrade: Institut zapsihologiju.

5 Pelowski, M., Markey, P.S., Forster, M., Gerger, G., & Leder, H. (2017). Move me, astonish me...delight my eyes and brain: The Vienna

Integrated Model of top-down and bottom-up processes in Art Perception (VIMAP) and corresponding affective, evaluative, and neurophysiological correlates. *Physics of Life Reviews, 21*, 80–125.

6 Cupchik, G.C., & Winston, A.S. (1996). Confluence and divergence in empirical aesthetics, philosophy, and mainstream psychology. In *Handbook of perception and cognition: Cognitive ecology*, 61–85.

7 Daykin, N., Byrne, E., Soteriou, T., & O'Connor, S. (2008). The impact of art, design and environment in mental healthcare: A systematic review of the literature. *Journal of the Royal Society for the Promotion of Health, 128*(2), 85–94; Silvia, P.J. (2005). Emotional responses to art: From collation and arousal to cognition and emotion. *Review of General Psychology, 9*(4), 342–357; Todd, C., Camic, P.M., Lockyer, B., Thomson, L.J., & Chatterjee, H.J. (2017). Museum-based programs for socially isolated older adults: Understanding what works. *Health & Place, 48*, 47–55.

8 Seligman, M.E. (2011). *Flourish: A visionary new understanding of happiness and well-being*. New York: Simon and Schuster.

9 Pawelski, J.O. (2016a). Defining the "positive" in positive psychology: Part I. A descriptive analysis. *Journal of Positive Psychology, 11*(4), 339–356; Pawelski, J.O. (2016b). Defining the "positive" in positive psychology: Part II. A normative analysis. *Journal of Positive Psychology, 11*(4), 357–365.

10 Leder, H., Belke, B., Oeberst, A., & Augustin, D. (2004). A model of aesthetic appreciation and aesthetic judgments. *British Journal of Psychology, 95*(4), 489–508; Zeki, S. (2001). Artistic creativity and the brain. *Science, 293*(5527), 51–52.

11 Konecni, V.J. (2010). Aesthetic trinity theory and the sublime. Proceedings of the European Society for Aesthetics, 2, 244–264; Schindler, I., Hosoya, G., Menninghaus, W., Beermann, U., Wagner, V., Eid, M., & Scherer, K.R. (2017). Measuring aesthetic emotions: A review of the literature and a new assessment tool. PLoS One, 12(6), e0178899.

12 Menninghaus, W., Wagner, V., Wassiliwizky, E., Schindler, I., Hanich, J., Jacobsen, T., & Koelsch, S. (2019). What are aesthetic emotions? *Psychological Review, 126*(2), 171.

13 Chirico, A., Clewis, R.R., Yaden, D.B., & Gaggioli, A. (2021). Nature versus art as elicitors of the sublime: A virtual reality study. *PloS One, 16*(3), e0233628; Clewis, R.R., Yaden, D.B., & Chirico, A. (2022). Intersections between awe and the sublime: A preliminary empirical study. *Empirical Studies of the Arts, 40*(2), 143–173.

14 Keltner, D., & Haidt, J. (2003). Approaching awe, a moral, spiritual, and aesthetic emotion. *Cognition and Emotion, 17*(2), 297–314.

15 Konečni, V.J. (2008). Does music induce emotion? A theoretical and methodological analysis. *Psychology of Aesthetics, Creativity, and the Arts, 2*(2), 115; Menninghaus, W., Wagner, V., Hanich, J., Wassiliwizky, E., Jacobsen, T., & Koelsch, S. (2017). The distancing-embracing model of the enjoyment of negative emotions in art reception. *Behavioral and Brain Sciences, 40,* e347.

16 Guan, F., Chen, J., Chen, O., Liu, L., & Zha, Y. (2019). Awe and prosocial tendency. Current Psychology, 38, 1033–1041; Piff, P.K., Dietze, P., Feinberg, M., Stancato, D.M., & Keltner, D. (2015). Awe, the small self, and prosocial behavior. Journal of Personality and Social Psychology, 108(6), 883; Shiota, M.N., Keltner, D., & Mossman, A. (2007). The nature of awe: Elicitors, appraisals, and effects on self-concept. Cognition and Emotion, 21(5), 944–963.

17 Silvia, P.J. (2013). Interested experts, confused novices: Art expertise and the knowledge emotions. Empirical Studies of the Arts, 31(1), 107–115; Silvia, P.J., & Nusbaum, E.C. (2011). On personality and piloerection: Individual differences in aesthetic chills and other unusual aesthetic experiences. Psychology of Aesthetics, Creativity, and the Arts, 5(3), 208.

18 Chamorro-Premuzic, T., Reimers, S., Hsu, A., & Ahmetoglu, G. (2009). Who art thou? Personality predictors of artistic preferences in a large UK sample: The importance of openness. *British Journal of Psychology, 100*(3), 501–516.

19 Ishizu, T., & Zeki, S. (2011). Toward a brain-based theory of beauty. *PLoS One, 6*(7), e21852.

20 Chatterjee, A., & Vartanian, O. (2016). Neuroscience of aesthetics. *Annals of the New York Academy of Sciences, 1369*(1), 172–194.

21 Vessel, E.A., Starr, G.G., & Rubin, N. (2012). The brain on art: Intense aesthetic experience activates the default mode network. *Frontiers in Human Neuroscience, 6,* 66.

22 Pilgrim, L., Norris, J.I., & Hackathorn, J. (2017). Music is awesome: Influences of emotion, personality, and preference on experienced awe. *Journal of Consumer Behaviour, 16*(5), 442–451.

23 Sachs, M.E., Damasio, A., & Habibi, A. (2015). The pleasures of sad music: A systematic review. *Frontiers in Human Neuroscience, 9,* 404.

24 Salimpoor, V.N., Zald, D.H., Zatorre, R.J., Dagher, A., & McIntosh, A.R. (2015). Predictions and the brain: How musical sounds become rewarding. *Trends in Cognitive Sciences, 19*(2), 86–91.

25 Cross, E.S., & Elizarova, A. (2014). Motor control in action: Using dance to explore the intricate choreography between action perception and production in the human brain. *Advances in Experimental Medicine and Biology,* 147–160.

26 Csikszentmihalyi, M. (2018). *Flow: The psychology of optimal experience by Mihaly Csikszentmihalyi.* Createspace Independent Publishing Platform. Retrieved from https://books.google.com/books?id=tSD3tgEACAAJ

27 Ikard, C.F. (2016). The Aesthetic experience, flow, and smart technology: Viewing art in a virtual environment (PhD diss., Walden University); Wanzer, D.L., Finley, K.P., Zarian, S., & Cortez, N. (2020). Experiencing flow while viewing art: Development of the aesthetic experience questionnaire. Psychology of Aesthetics, Creativity, and the Arts, 14(1), 113.

28 Chilton, G. (2013). Art therapy and flow: A review of the literature and applications. Art Therapy, 30(2), 64–70; Wrigley, W.J., & Emmerson, S.B. (2013). The experience of the flow state in live music performance. Psychology of Music, 41(3), 292–305.

29 Im, S., & Varma, S. (2018). Distorted time perception during flow as revealed by an attention-demanding cognitive task. *Creativity Research Journal, 30*(3), 295–304.

30 Jackson, S.A., & Marsh, H.W. (1996). Development and validation of a scale to measure optimal experience: The Flow State Scale. Journal of Sport and Exercise Psychology, 18(1), 17–35; Nakamura, J., & Csikszentmihalyi, M. (2009). Flow theory and research. Handbook of Positive Psychology, 195, 206.

31 Cseh, G.M., Phillips, L.H., & Pearson, D G. (2015). Flow, affect and visual creativity. Cognition and Emotion, 29(2), 281–291; Dan, Y. (2021). Examining the relationships between learning interest, flow, and creativity. School Psychology International, 42(2), 157–169.

32 Fullagar, C.J., Knight, P.A., & Sovern, H S. (2013). Challenge/skill balance, flow, and performance anxiety. *Applied Psychology, 62*(2), 236–259; Harris, D.J., Allen, K.L., Vine, S.J., & Wilson, M.R. (2023). A systematic review and meta-analysis of the relationship between flow

states and performance. *International Review of Sport and Exercise Psychology, 16*(1), 693–721.

33 Csikszentmihalyi, M. (2018). *Flow: The psychology of optimal experience by Mihaly Csikszentmihalyi.* CreateSpace Independent Publishing Platform. Retrieved from https://books.google.com/books?id=tSD3tgEACAAJ

34 Macdonald, A.S. (2002). The scenario of sensory encounter: Cultural factors in sensory—Aesthetic experience. In *Pleasure with products: Beyond usability*, 109–119. London: Taylor & Francis.

35 Fu, Y.-N., Feng, R., Liu, Q., He, Y., Turel, O., Zhang, S., & He, Q. (2022). Awe and prosocial behavior: The mediating role of presence of meaning in life and the moderating role of perceived social support. International Journal of Environmental Research and Public Health, 19(11), 6466; Guan, F., Chen, J., Chen, O., Liu, L., & Zha, Y. (2019). Awe and prosocial tendency. Current Psychology, 38, 1033–1041; Piff, P.K., Dietze, P., Feinberg, M., Stancato, D.M., & Keltner, D. (2015). Awe, the small self, and prosocial behavior. Journal of Personality and Social Psychology, 108(6), 883.

36 Graziosi, M., & Yaden, D. (2021). Interpersonal awe: Exploring the social domain of awe elicitors. *Journal of Positive Psychology, 16*(2), 263–271.

37 Kou, X., Konrath, S., & Goldstein, T.R. (2020). The relationship among different types of arts engagement, empathy, and prosocial behavior. *Psychology of Aesthetics, Creativity, and the Arts, 14*(4), 481.

38 Shim, Y., Tay, L., Ward, M., & Pawelski, J.O. (2019). Arts and humanities engagement: An integrative conceptual framework for psychological research. *Review of General Psychology, 23*(2), 159–176.

39 Archer, L., Dawson, E., DeWitt, J., Seakins, A., & Wong, B. (2015). "Science capital": A conceptual, methodological, and empirical argument for extending bourdieusian notions of capital beyond the arts. *Journal of Research in Science Teaching, 52*(7), 922–948.

40 Coulangeon, P., & Lemel, Y. (2009). Cultural and sports participation in France: Choices, diversity, and accumulation. *Economie & Statistique.*

41 Milne, C., & Otieno, T. (2007). Understanding engagement: Science demonstrations and emotional energy. *Science Education, 91*(4), 523–553.

42　Piff, P.K., Dietze, P., Feinberg, M., Stancato, D.M., & Keltner, D. (2015). Awe, the small self, and prosocial behavior. *Journal of Personality and Social Psychology*, *108*(6), 883.

43　O'Brien, D. (2010). *Measuring the value of culture: A report to the Department for Culture, Media and Sport*. Leeds Metropolitan University.

44　Vessel, E.A., Starr, G.G., & Rubin, N. (2012). The brain on art: Intense aesthetic experience activates the default mode network. *Frontiers in Human Neuroscience*, 6, 66.

45　Molenberghs, P., Cunnington, R., & Mattingley, J.B. (2012). Brain regions with mirror properties: A meta-analysis of 125 human fMRI studies. *Neuroscience & Biobehavioral Reviews*, *36*(1), 341–349; Rizzolatti, G., & Craighero, L. (2004). The mirror-neuron system. *Annual Review of Neuroscience*, *27*, 169–192.

46　Di Pellegrino, G., Fadiga, L., Fogassi, L., Gallese, V., & Rizzolatti, G. (1992). Understanding motor events: A neurophysiological study. *Experimental Brain Research*, *91*, 176–180; Gallese, V., Fadiga, L., Fogassi, L., & Rizzolatti, G. (1996). Action recognition in the pre-motor cortex. *Brain*, *119*(2), 593–609.

47　Nummenmaa, L., Hirvonen, J., Parkkola, R., & Hietanen, J.K. (2008). Is emotional contagion special? An fMRI study on neural systems for affective and cognitive empathy. *Neuroimage*, *43*(3), 571–580.

48　Christov-Moore, L., Simpson, E.A., Coudé, G., Grigaityte, K., Iacoboni, M., & Ferrari, P.F. (2014). Empathy: Gender effects in brain and behavior. *Neuroscience & Biobehavioral Reviews*, *46*, 604–627.

49　Seligman, M.E. (2011). *Flourish: A visionary new understanding of happiness and well-being*. New York: Simon & Schuster.

50　Chirico, A., Serafini, F., Pizzolante, M., Malvezzi, R., Gianotti, E., Micucci, C., et al. (2022). Inspiring awe in high school teachers: Design and preliminary test of a virtual training on AltspaceVR. *Annual Review of Cybertherapy and Telemedicine*, 20(A), 14.

51　Pelowski, M., & Akiba, F. (2011). A model of art perception, evaluation and emotion in transformative aesthetic experience. *New Ideas in Psychology*, *29*(2), 80–97.

52　Funch, B.S. (2021). Art, emotion, and existential well-being. *Journal of Theoretical and Philosophical Psychology*, *41*(1), 5; Lasher, M.D., Carroll, J.M., & Bever, T.G. (1983). The cognitive basis of aesthetic experience. *Leonardo*, 196–199; Neuhofer, B., Celuch, K., & To, T.L. (2020). Experience design and the dimensions of transformative festival experiences. *International Journal of Contemporary Hospitality Management, 32*(9), 2881–2901.

53 Pelowski, M., Markey, P.S., Forster, M., Gerger, G., & Leder, H. (2017). Move me, astonish me…delight my eyes and brain: The Vienna Integrated Model of top-down and bottom-up processes in Art Perception (VIMAP) and corresponding affective, evaluative, and neurophysiological correlates. *Physics of Life Reviews, 21*, 80–125.

54 Pelowski, M., Markey, P.S., Forster, M., Gerger, G., & Leder, H. (2017). Move me, astonish me…delight my eyes and brain: The Vienna Integrated Model of top-down and bottom-up processes in Art Perception (VIMAP) and corresponding affective, evaluative, and neurophysiological correlates. *Physics of Life Reviews, 21*, 80–125.

55 Pelowski, M. (2015). Tears and transformation: Feeling like crying as an indicator of insightful or "aesthetic" experience with art. *Frontiers in Psychology, 6*, 1006.

56 Seligman, M.E. (2002). *Authentic happiness: Using the new positive psychology to realize your potential for lasting fulfillment.* New York: Simon & Schuster.)

57 Hennessey, B.A., & Amabile, T.M. (1987). *Creativity and learning: What research says to the teacher.* ERIC.

58 Leder, H., Mitrovic, A., & Goller, J. (2016). How beauty determines gaze! Facial attractiveness and gaze duration in images of real-world scenes. *I-Perception, 7*(4), 2041669516664355.

59 Cupchik, G.C., & Winston, A.S. (1996). Confluence and divergence in empirical aesthetics, philosophy, and mainstream psychology. In *Handbook of perception and cognition: Cognitive ecology*, 61–85.

60 Bolwerk, A., Mack-Andrick, J., Lang, F.R., Dörfler, A., & Maihöfner, C. (2014). How art changes your brain: Differential effects of visual art production and cognitive art evaluation on functional brain connectivity. *PLoS One, 9*(7), e101035.

61 Winner, E., & Hetland, L. (2000). The arts in education: Evaluating the evidence for a causal link. *Journal of Aesthetic Education*, 3–10.

62 Chan, S.C., Chan, C.C., Derbie, A.Y., Hui, I., Tan, D.G., Pang, M.Y., Lau, S.C., & Fong, K.N. (2017). Chinese calligraphy writing for augmenting attentional control and working memory of older

adults at risk of mild cognitive impairment: A randomized controlled trial. *Journal of Alzheimer's Disease, 58*(3), 735–746.

63 Hanna-Pladdy, B., & MacKay, A. (2011). The relation between instrumental musical activity and cognitive aging. *Neuropsychology, 25*(3), 378.

64 Pinho, A.L., de Manzano, Ö., Fransson, P., Eriksson, H., & Ullén, F. (2014). Connecting to create: Expertise in musical improvisation is associated with increased functional connectivity between premotor and prefrontal areas. *Journal of Neuroscience, 34*(18), 6156–6163.

65 World Health Organization. (2021). *Arts and health.* Retrieved from https://www.who.int/initiatives/arts-and-health; World Health Organization. (2023). *The power of healing: New WHO report shows how arts can help beat noncommunicable diseases.* Retrieved from https://www.who.int/europe/news/item/15-11-2023-the-power-of-healing--new-who-report-shows-how-arts-can-help-beat-noncommunicable-diseases

66 National Endowment for the Arts. (2020). Arts and health. Retrieved from https://www.arts.gov/impact/arts-and-health

67 Dalley, T. (2008). Art as therapy: An introduction to the use of art as a therapeutic technique. Routledge; Fancourt, D., Steptoe, A., & Cadar, D. (2018). Cultural engagement and cognitive reserve: Museum attendance and dementia incidence over a 10-year period. *British Journal of Psychiatry, 213*(5), 661–663.

68 Skov, M., & Nadal, M. (2023). Can arts-based interventions improve health? A conceptual and methodological critique of art therapy. doi:10.31234/osf.io/sp9y3; Aspen Institute. (2021). *NeuroArts blueprint. Advancing the science of arts, health, and wellbeing* (32). Retrieved from. https://neuroartsblueprint.org/wp-content/uploads/2021/11/NeuroArtsBlue_ExSumReport_FinalOnline_spreads_v32.pdf

69 Malchiodi, C.A. (2012). Introduction to art therapy in health care settings. *Art Therapy and Health Care*, 1–12.

70 Stuckey, H.L., & Nobel, J. (2010). The connection between art, healing, and public health: A review of current literature. *American Journal of Public Health, 100*(2), 254–263.

71 Malchiodi, C.A. (2012). Introduction to art therapy in health care settings. Art Therapy and Health Care, 1–12; Van Lith, T., & Beerse, M.

(2019). Examination of contemporary and promising research strategies in art therapy. Art Therapy, 36(3), 141–148.

72 Fancourt, D., & Finn, S. (2019). *What is the evidence on the role of the arts in improving health and well-being? A scoping review.* World Health Organization. Regional Office for Europe.

73 Monti, D.A., Peterson, C., Kunkel, E.J.S., Hauck, W.W., Pequignot, E., Rhodes, L., & Brainard, G.C. (2006). A randomized, controlled trial of mindfulness-based art therapy (MBAT) for women with cancer. *Psycho-Oncology: Journal of the Psychological, Social and Behavioral Dimensions of Cancer, 15*(5), 363–373.

74 Newland, P., & Bettencourt, B.A. (2020). Effectiveness of mindfulness-based art therapy for symptoms of anxiety, depression, and fatigue: A systematic review and meta-analysis. *Complementary Therapies in Clinical Practice, 41*, 101246.

75 Hillecke, T., Nickel, A., & Bolay, H.V. (2005). Scientific perspectives on music therapy. *Annals of the New York Academy of Sciences, 1060*(1), 271–282; Peters, J.S. (1987). *Music therapy: An introduction.* Charles C Thomas.

76 Gold, C., Solli, H.P., Krüger, V., & Lie, S.A. (2009). Dose–response relationship in music therapy for people with serious mental disorders: Systematic review and meta-analysis. *Clinical Psychology Review, 29*(3), 193–207.

77 Bradt, J., Dileo, C., Magill, L., & Teague, A. (2016). Music interventions for improving psychological and physical outcomes in cancer patients. *Cochrane Database of Systematic Reviews, 8*. Retrieved from https://www.cochranelibrary.com/cdsr/doi/10.1002/14651858. CD006911.pub3/abstract

78 Tang, Q., Huang, Z., Zhou, H., & Ye, P. (2020). Effects of music therapy on depression: A meta-analysis of randomized controlled trials. *PLoS One, 15*(11), e0240862.

79 Chan, M.F., Chung, Y.F.L., Chung, S.W.A., & Lee, O.K.A. (2009). Investigating the physiological responses of patients listening to music in the intensive care unit. *Journal of Clinical Nursing, 18*(9), 1250–1257; Raglio, A., Galandra, C., Sibilla, L., Esposito, F., Gaeta, F., Di Salle, F., Moro, L., Carne, I., Bastianello, S., & Baldi, M. (2016). Effects of active music therapy on the normal brain: fMRI based evidence. *Brain Imaging and Behavior, 10*, 182–186.

80 Nilsson, U. (2008). The anxiety-and pain-reducing effects of music interventions: A systematic review. *AORN Journal*, *87*(4), 780–807.

81 Nilsson, U., Unosson, M., & Rawal, N. (2005). Stress reduction and analgesia in patients exposed to calming music postoperatively: A randomized controlled trial. *European Journal of Anaesthesiology*, *22*(2), 96–102.

82 Guetin, S., Portet, F., Picot, M., Pommié, C., Messaoudi, M., Djabelkir, L., Olsen, A., Cano, M., Lecourt, E., & Touchon, J. (2009). Effect of music therapy on anxiety and depression in patients with Alzheimer's type dementia: Randomised, controlled study. *Dementia and Geriatric Cognitive Disorders*, *28*(1), 36–46.

83 Silverman, M.J. (2019). Quantitative comparison of group-based music therapy experiences in an acute care adult mental health setting: A four-group cluster-randomized study. *Nordic Journal of Music Therapy*, *28*(1), 41–59.

84 Wang, L., Peng, J., Xiang, W., Huang, Y., & Chen, A. (2022). Effects of rhythmic auditory stimulation on motor function and balance ability in stroke: A systematic review and meta-analysis of clinical randomized controlled studies. *Frontiers in Neuroscience*, *16*, 1043575.

85 Corazon, S.S., Sidenius, U., Poulsen, D.V., Gramkow, M.C., & Stigsdotter, U.K. (2019). Psycho-physiological stress recovery in outdoor nature-based interventions: A systematic review of the past eight years of research. *International Journal of Environmental Research and Public Health*, *16*(10), 1711; Silva, A., Matos, M., & Gonçalves, M. (2023). Nature and human well-being: A systematic review of empirical evidence from nature-based interventions. *Journal of Environmental Planning and Management*, 1–58.

86 Ulrich, R.S. (1984). View through a window may influence recovery from surgery. *Science*, *224*(4647), 420–421.

87 Park, S.-H., & Mattson, R.H. (2008). Effects of flowering and foliage plants in hospital rooms on patients recovering from abdominal surgery. *HortTechnology*, *18*(4), 563–568; Park, S.-H., & Mattson, R.H. (2009). Therapeutic influences of plants in hospital rooms on surgical recovery. *HortScience*, *44*(1), 102–105.

88 Berman, M.G., Kross, E., Krpan, K.M., Askren, M.K., Burson, A., Deldin, P.J., Kaplan, S., Sherdell, L., Gotlib, I.H., & Jonides, J. (2012). Interacting

with nature improves cognition and affect for individuals with depression. *Journal of Affective Disorders*, *140*(3), 300–305.

89 Jones, R., Tarter, R., & Ross, A.M. (2021). Greenspace interventions, stress and cortisol: A scoping review. *International Journal of Environmental Research and Public Health*, *18*(6), 2802. https://doi.org/10.3390/ijerph18062802

90 Hartig, T., Mitchell, R., de Vries, S., & Frumkin, H. (2014). Nature and health. *Annual Review of Public Health*, *35*(1), 207–228. https://doi.org/10.1146/annurev-publhealth-032013-182443

91 Bratman, G.N., Daily, G.C., Levy, B.J., & Gross, J.J. (2015). The benefits of nature experience: Improved affect and cognition. *Landscape and Urban Planning*, *138*, 41–50. https://doi.org/10.1016/j.landurbplan.2015.02.005

92 Annerstedt, M., & Währborg, P. (2011). Nature-assisted therapy: Systematic review of controlled and observational studies. *Scandinavian Journal of Public Health*, *39*(4), 371–388. https://doi.org/10.1177/1403494810396400

93 Annerstedt, M., Jönsson, P., Wallergård, M., Johansson, G., Karlson, B., Grahn, P., Hansen, Å.M., & Währborg, P. (2013). Inducing physiological stress recovery with sounds of nature in a virtual reality forest—Results from a pilot study. *Physiology & Behavior*, *118*, 240–250. https://doi.org/10.1016/j.physbeh.2013.05.023

94 Poulsen, D.V., Stigsdotter, U.K., & Refshage, A.D. (2015). Whatever happened to the soldiers? Nature-assisted therapies for veterans diagnosed with post-traumatic stress disorder: A literature review. *Urban Forestry & Urban Greening*, *14*(2), 438–445. https://doi.org/10.1016/j.ufug.2015.03.009

95 Poulsen, D.V., Stigsdotter, U.K., & Refshage, A.D. (2015). Whatever happened to the soldiers? Nature-assisted therapies for veterans diagnosed with post-traumatic stress disorder: A literature review. *Urban Forestry & Urban Greening*, *14*(2), 438–445. https://doi.org/10.1016/j.ufug.2015.03.009

96 Anderson, C.L., Monroy, M., & Keltner, D. (2018). Awe in nature heals: Evidence from military veterans, at-risk youth, and college students. *Emotion*, *18*(8), 1195

97 Meekums, B. (2002). Dance movement therapy: A creative psychotherapeutic approach. *Dance Movement Therapy*, 1–130.

98 Payne, H., Warnecke, T., Karkou, V., & Westland, G. (2016). A comparative analysis of body psychotherapy and dance movement psychotherapy from a European perspective. *Body, Movement and Dance in Psychotherapy, 11*(2–3), 144–166.

99 Savidaki, M., Demirtoka, S., & Rodríguez-Jiménez, R.M. (2020). Re-inhabiting one's body: A pilot study on the effects of dance movement therapy on body image and alexithymia in eating disorders. *Journal of Eating Disorders, 8,* 22. https://doi.org/10.1186/s40337-010-00296-2

100 Meekums, B. (2002). Dance movement therapy: A creative psycho-therapeutic approach. *Dance Movement Therapy,* 1–130.

101 Payne, H., Warnecke, T., Karkou, V., & Westland, G. (2016). A comparative analysis of body psychotherapy and dance movement psychotherapy from a European perspective. *Body, Movement and Dance in Psychotherapy, 11*(2–3), 144–166.

102 Wang, K. (2023). The effectiveness of using dance/movement therapy as a complementary and alternative medicine in palliative care and hospice care: A systematic literature review (PhD diss., Pratt Institute); Bradt, J., Shim, M., & Goodill, S.W. (2015). Dance/movement therapy for improving psychological and physical outcomes in cancer patients. *Cochrane Database of Systematic Reviews,* 1.

103 Payne, H., Warnecke, T., Karkou, V., & Westland, G. (2016). A comparative analysis of body psychotherapy and dance movement psychotherapy from a European perspective. *Body, Movement and Dance in Psychotherapy, 11*(2–3), 144–166; Wang, K. (2023). The effectiveness of using dance/movement therapy as a complementary and alternative medicine in Palliative Care and Hospice Care: A systematic literature review (PhD diss., Pratt Institute).

104 Burns, A. (2016). The effect of dance movement therapy on the self-esteem and state of hostility of sexually abused adolescents at a children's home. Retrieved from https://repository.up.ac.za/handle/2263/57229

105 Payne, H., Warnecke, T., Karkou, V., & Westland, G. (2016). A comparative analysis of body psychotherapy and dance movement psychotherapy from a European perspective. *Body, Movement and Dance in Psychotherapy, 11*(2–3), 144–166.

106 Yaden, D.B., Eichstaedt, J.C., & Medaglia, J.D. (2018). The future of technology in positive psychology: Methodological advances in the science of well-being. *Frontiers in Psychology*, *9*, 962.

107 Riva, G., Davide, F., & IJsselsteijn, W.A. (2003). Being there: The experience of presence in mediated environments. In *Being there: Concepts, effects and measurement of user presence in synthetic environments*, *5*; Slater, M. (2009). Place illusion and plausibility can lead to realistic behaviour in immersive virtual environments. *Philosophical Transactions of the Royal Society B: Biological Sciences*, *364*(1535), 3549–3557; Slater, M., & Sanchez-Vives, M.V. (2016). Enhancing our lives with immersive virtual reality. *Frontiers in Robotics and AI*, *3*, 74.

108 See, for example, Botella, C., Baños, R.M., García-Palacios, A., & Quero, S. (2017). Virtual reality and other realities. In *The science of cognitive behavioral therapy*, 551–590. Elsevier; Gaggioli, A., Villani, D., Serino, S., Banos, R., & Botella, C. (2019). Positive technology: Designing e-experiences for positive change. *Frontiers in Psychology*, *10*, 1571; Riva, G., Baños, R.M., Botella, C., Wiederhold, B.K., & Gaggioli, A. (2012). Positive technology: Using interactive technologies to promote positive functioning. *Cyberpsychology, Behavior, and Social Networking*, *15*(2), 69–77.

109 Riva, G., Baños, R.M., Botella, C., Mantovani, F., & Gaggioli, A. (2016). Transforming experience: The potential of augmented reality and virtual reality for enhancing personal and clinical change. *Frontiers in Psychiatry*, *7*, 164.

110 Riva, G. (1998). Virtual environments in neuroscience. *IEEE Transactions on Information Technology in Biomedicine*, *2*(4), 275–281.

111 Riva, G., Baños, R.M., Botella, C., Mantovani, F., & Gaggioli, A. (2016). Transforming experience: The potential of augmented reality and virtual reality for enhancing personal and clinical change. *Frontiers in Psychiatry*, *7*, 164; Vincelli, F. (1999). From imagination to virtual reality: The future of clinical psychology. *CyberPsychology and Behavior*, *2*(3), 241–248; Vincelli, F., Molinari, E., & Riva, G. (2001). Virtual reality as clinical tool: Immersion and three-dimensionality in the relationship between patient and therapist. In *Medicine meets virtual reality 2001*, 551–553. IOS Press.

112 Marco, J.H., Perpiñá, C., & Botella, C. (2013). Effectiveness of cognitive behavioral therapy supported by virtual reality in the treatment

of body image in eating disorders: One year follow-up. *Psychiatry Research*, *209*(3), 619–625; Perpiñá, C., Botella, C., & Baños, R. (2003). Virtual reality in eating disorders. *European Eating Disorders Review*, *11*(3), 261–278.

113 Falconer, C.J., Rovira, A., King, J.A., Gilbert, P., Antley, A., Fearon, P., Ralph, N., Slater, M., & Brewin, C.R. (2016). Embodying self-compassion within virtual reality and its effects on patients with depression. *BJPsych Open*, *2*(1), 74–80; Fodor, L.A., Coteţ, C.D., Cuijpers, P., Szamoskozi, Ş., David, D., & Cristea, I.A. (2018). The effectiveness of virtual reality-based interventions for symptoms of anxiety and depression: A meta-analysis. *Scientific Reports*, *8*(1), 10323.

114 Bouchard, S., Dumoulin, S., Robillard, G., Guitard, T., Klinger, E., Forget, H., Loranger, C., & Roucaut, F.X. (2017). Virtual reality compared with in vivo exposure in the treatment of social anxiety disorder: A three-arm randomised controlled trial. *British Journal of Psychiatry*, *210*(4), 276–283; Gorini, A., & Riva, G. (2008). Virtual reality in anxiety disorders: The past and the future. *Expert Review of Neurotherapeutics*, *8*(2), 215–233; Powers, M.B., & Emmelkamp, P.M. (2008). Virtual reality exposure therapy for anxiety disorders: A meta-analysis. *Journal of Anxiety Disorders*, *22*(3), 561–569.

115 Lam, P., Hebert, D., Boger, J., Lacheray, H., Gardner, D., Apkarian, J., & Mihailidis, A. (2008). A haptic-robotic platform for upper-limb reaching stroke therapy: Preliminary design and evaluation results. *Journal of NeuroEngineering and Rehabilitation*, *5*(1), 1–13; Laver, K. (2020). Virtual reality for stroke rehabilitation. In *Virtual reality in health and rehabilitation*, 19–28. CRC Press.

116 Enrique, Á., Bretón-López, J., Molinari, G., Baños, R.M., & Botella, C. (2018). Efficacy of an adaptation of the Best Possible Self intervention implemented through positive technology: A randomized control trial. *Applied Research in Quality of Life*, *13*, 671–689.

117 Wiederhold, B.K., Gao, K., Sulea, C., & Wiederhold, M.D. (2014). Virtual reality as a distraction technique in chronic pain patients. *Cyberpsychology, Behavior, and Social Networking*, *17*(6), 346–352.

118 Rothbaum, B.O., Hodges, L.F., Ready, D., Graap, K., & Alarcon, R.D. (2001). Virtual reality exposure therapy for Vietnam veterans with posttraumatic stress disorder. *Journal of Clinical Psychiatry*, *62*(8), 617–622.

119 Gold, C., Solli, H.P., Krüger, V., & Lie, S.A. (2009). Dose–response relationship in music therapy for people with serious mental disorders: Systematic review and meta-analysis. *Clinical Psychology Review*, *29*(3), 193–207; Gold, J.I., & Mahrer, N.E. (2018). Is virtual reality ready for prime time in the medical space? A randomized control trial of pediatric virtual reality for acute procedural pain management. *Journal of Pediatric Psychology*, *43*(3), 266–275.

120 Colombo, D., Díaz-García, A., Fernandez-Álvarez, J., & Botella, C. (2021). Virtual reality for the enhancement of emotion regulation. *Clinical Psychology & Psychotherapy*, *28*(3), 519–537; Colombo, D., Fernández-Álvarez, J., Garcia Palacios, A., Cipresso, P., Botella, C., & Riva, G. (2019). New technologies for the understanding, assessment, and intervention of emotion regulation. *Frontiers in Psychology*, *10*, 1261; Montana, J.I., Matamala-Gomez, M., Maisto, M., Mavrodiev, P.A., Cavalera, C.M., Diana, B., Mantovani, F., & Realdon, O. (2020). The benefits of emotion regulation interventions in virtual reality for the improvement of wellbeing in adults and older adults: A systematic review. *Journal of Clinical Medicine*, *9*(2), 500.

121 Schutte, N.S., & Stilinović, E.J. (2017). Facilitating empathy through virtual reality. *Motivation and Emotion*, *41*, 708–712; Shin, D. (2018). Empathy and embodied experience in virtual environment: To what extent can virtual reality stimulate empathy and embodied experience? *Computers in Human Behavior*, *78*, 64–73; Ventura, S., Badenes-Ribera, L., Herrero, R., Cebolla, A., Galiana, L., & Baños, R. (2020). Virtual reality as a medium to elicit empathy: A meta-analysis. *Cyberpsychology, Behavior, and Social Networking*, *23*(10), 667–676.

122 Chirico, A., Glaveanu, V.P., Cipresso, P., Riva, G., & Gaggioli, A. (2018). Awe enhances creative thinking: An experimental study. Creativity Research Journal, 30(2), 123–131; Chirico, A., Serafini, F., Pizzolante, M., Malvezzi, R., Gianotti, E., Micucci, C., et al. (2022). Inspiring awe in high school teachers: Design and preliminary test of a virtual training on AltspaceVR. Annual Review of Cybertherapy and Telemedicine, 20(A), 31–35; Chirico, A., Pizzolante, M., Borghesi, F., Bartolotta, S., Sarcinella, E.D., Cipresso, P., & Gaggioli, A. (2023). "Standing up for earth rights": Awe-inspiring virtual nature for promoting pro-environmental behaviors. Cyberpsychology, Behavior, and Social Networking, 26(4), 300–308; Quesnel, D., & Riecke, B.E. (2018). Are you awed yet? How virtual reality gives us awe

and goose bumps. Frontiers in Psychology, 9, 2158; Pizzolante, M., Sarcinella, E.D., Borghesi, F., Bartolotta, S., Gaggioli, A., & Chirico, A. (2023). " Being immersed in aesthetic emotions": Comparing immersive Vs. Non immersive VR in aesthetic emotions elicitation. Annual Review of Cybertherapy and Telemedicine, 21(A), 117–123.

123 Stepanova, E.R., Quesnel, D., & Riecke, B.E. (2019). Space—A virtual frontier: How to design and evaluate a virtual reality experience of the overview effect. *Frontiers in Digital Humanities*, 6, 7.

124 Yaden, D.B., Iwry, J., Slack, K J., Eichstaedt, J.C., Zhao, Y., Vaillant, G.E., & Newberg, A.B. (2016). The overview effect: Awe and self-transcendent experience in space flight. *Psychology of Consciousness: Theory, Research, and Practice*, 3(1), 1.

125 Anadol, R. (2018). Melting Memories. *Art* Charles C Thomas Retrieved May 3, 2019.

126 Diodato, R. (2022). Virtual reality and aesthetic experience. *Philosophies*, 7(2), 29; Kwastek, K. (2016). Immersed in reflection? The aesthetic experience of interactive media art. In *Immersion in the visual arts and media*, 66–85. Brill; Gere, C. (2008). New media art and the gallery in the digital age. In *New media in the white cube and beyond: Curatorial models for digital art*, 13–25; Iosa, M., Bini, F., Marinozzi, F., Antonucci, G., Pascucci, S., Baghini, G., Guarino, V., Paolucci, S., Morone, G., & Tieri, G. (2022). Inside the Michelangelo effect: The role of art and aesthetic attractiveness on perceived fatigue and hand kinematics in virtual painting. *PsyCh Journal*, 11(5), 748–754; Trupp, M.D., Bignardi, G., Specker, E., Vessel, E.A., & Pelowski, M. (2023). Who benefits from online art viewing, and how: The role of pleasure, meaningfulness, and trait aesthetic responsiveness in computer-based art interventions for well-being. *Computers in Human Behavior*, 145, 107764.

127 Marín-Morales, J., Higuera-Trujillo, J., Greco, A., Guixeres, J., Llinares, C., Gentili, C., Scilingo, E., Alcañiz, M., & Valenza, G. (2019). Real vs. immersive-virtual emotional experience: Analysis of psycho-physiological patterns in a free exploration of an art museum. *PLoS One*, 14.

128 Chirico, A., & Gaggioli, A. (2021). The potential role of awe for depression: Reassembling the puzzle. *Frontiers in Psychology*, 12, 617715.

129 Slater, M., & Wilbur, S. (1997). A framework for immersive virtual environments: Speculations on the role of presence in virtual

environments. *Presence: Teleoperators and Virtual Environments,* *6*(6),603–616.

130 Pizzolante, M., Sarcinella, E.D., Borghesi, F., Bartolotta, S., Gaggioli, A., & Chirico, A. (2023). " Being Immersed in Aesthetic Emotions": Comparing immersive Vs. Non immersive VR in Aesthetic Emotions Elicitation. *Annual Review of Cybertherapy and Telemedicine, 21*(A), 117–123.

131 Lombard, M., & Ditton, T. (1997). At the heart of it all: The concept of presence. *Journal of Computer-Mediated Communication, 3*(2), JCMC321; Slater, M. (2003). A note on presence terminology. *Presence Connect, 3*(3),1–5.

132 Guazzaroni, G. (2020). Role of emotions in interactive museums: How art and virtual reality affect emotions. In *Virtual and augmented reality in education, art, and museums,* 174–193. IGI Global; Pizzolante, M., & Chirico, A. (2022). *"You Can Tell a Man by the Emotion He Feels": How emotions influence visual inspection of abstract art in immersive virtual reality,* 341–359. Berlin: Springer Verlag; Pizzolante, M., Sarcinella, E.D., Borghesi, F., Bartolotta, S., Gaggioli, A., & Chirico, A. (2023). Being immersed in aesthetic emotions: Comparing immersive vs. non-immersive VR in aesthetic emotions elicitation. *Annual Review of Cybertherapy and Telemedicine, 21*(A), 117–123.

133 Ulrich, R.S., Zimring, C., Zhu, X., DuBose, J., Seo, H.-B., Choi, Y.-S., Quan, X., & Joseph, A. (2008). A review of the research literature on evidence-based healthcare design. *HERD: Health Environments Research & Design Journal, 1*(3), 61–125.

134 Collie, K., & Čubranić, D. (2002). Computer-supported distance art therapy: A focus on traumatic illness. *Journal of Technology in Human Services, 20*(1–2), 155–171; Levy, C.E., Spooner, H., Lee, J.B., Sonke, J., Myers, K., & Snow, E. (2018). Telehealth-based creative arts therapy: Transforming mental health and rehabilitation care for rural veterans. *Arts in Psychotherapy, 57,* 20–26.

135 Barber, B., Brandoff, R., Lombardi, R., Carlton, N., Choe, N.S., Darke, K., Ehinger, J., Hall, K., Hsin, C., & L'Esperance, N. (2016). *Digital art therapy: Material, methods, and applications.* Jessica Kingsley; Hacmun, I., Regev, D., & Salomon, R. (2018). The principles of art therapy in virtual reality. *Frontiers in Psychology, 9,* 2082.

136 Bolton, R.N., McColl-Kennedy, J.R., Cheung, L., Gallan, A., Orsingher, C., Witell, L., & Zaki, M. (2018). Customer experience challenges: Bringing together digital, physical and social realms. *Journal of Service Management*, *29*(5), 776–808.

137 Rizzo, A., & Koenig, S.T. (2017). Is clinical virtual reality ready for primetime? *Neuropsychology*, *31*(8), 877.

138 Rizzo, A., & Koenig, S.T. (2017). Is clinical virtual reality ready for primetime? *Neuropsychology*, *31*(8), 877.

139 Pillai, A.S., & Mathew, P.S. (2019). Impact of virtual reality in healthcare: A review. *Virtual and Augmented Reality in Mental Health Treatment*, 17–31.

140 Wilson, C.J., & Soranzo, A. (2015). The use of virtual reality in psychology: A case study in visual perception. In *Computational and mathematical methods in medicine*.

141 Di Maria, A. (2019). *Exploring ethical dilemmas in art therapy: 50 clinicians from 20 countries share their stories*. Routledge.

142 Craske, M.G., Meuret, A.E., Ritz, T., Treanor, M., Dour, H., & Rosenfield, D. (2019). Positive affect treatment for depression and anxiety: A randomized clinical trial for a core feature of anhedonia. *Journal of Consulting and Clinical Psychology*, *87*(5), 457.

143 Moon, B.L., & Nolan, E.G. (2019). *Ethical issues in art therapy*. Charles C Thomas.

9

Skill Sets of the Facilitator

Kathleen D. Benton, Teri Yarbrow,
Nidhi A. Patel, and Erin Allen

Immersive VR Therapy and Its Uses

A virtual-reality (VR) therapist or immersive therapist is one who uses virtual-reality technology to immerse patients into fully digitally created synthetic worlds by using a head-mounted display (HMD). Immersive experiences using a VR headset have proven, measurable, and beneficial results with patients. Immersive VR therapy uses VR for patients in a great number of ways:

- ◆ Palliative care
- ◆ Pain management
- ◆ Children's pediatrics
- ◆ Spinal cord injuries
- ◆ Dementia and Alzheimer's
- ◆ Medical training and education
- ◆ Virtual surgical assist
- ◆ Hospice
- ◆ Elder care
- ◆ Stress relief

DOI: 10.4324/9781032649771-9

- Anxiety and depression
- Opioid addiction
- Drug rehab
- Pre-operative care
- Prenatal care
- Dental issues
- Physical therapy
- Phlebotomy
- Posttraumatic stress disorder (PTSD)
- Increasing empathy
- Labor and delivery pain
- Cognitive rehabilitation
- Stroke rehabilitation

VR immersive therapy is being successfully used across the nation in leading hospitals, health centers, and for in-home care. A recent survey found that 77% of healthcare organizations have implemented or plan to implement virtual-reality technology.[1] Currently, there are over 25 known institutions. Some of the many hospitals worldwide using VR are Cedars-Sinai Medical Center, the Mayo Clinic, Yale School of Medicine, and Harvard's School of Medicine.

After years of research and thousands of published articles, immersive reality experiences as therapy are now validated by the Federal Drug Administration (FDA). In 2021, the FDA gave this area a designation as MXR—Medical Extended Reality, which includes VR, augmented reality (AR), and mixed reality (MR).

In May 2023, the American Medical Extended Reality Association (AMXRA) was founded. "The mission of AMXRA is to advance the science and practice of medical extended reality through advancing care delivery, scientific investigation, innovation, education, advocacy, and community" (https://www.amxra.org). Just as the American Medical Association promotes the betterment of health and practices, AMXRA will create standards and practices for utilizing and delivering immersive reality therapy.

The Meaning Found in Spirituality and VR

Spirituality can be how patients learn to cope with processing disease. Many studies have been cited to identify how professionals and patients see spiritual needs. Common themes include the desire for positivity, feelings of peace and comfort, feelings of joy, and the need to receive meaning, hope, and gratitude. VR, when facilitated adequately, can initiate this healing.

A vast amount of all literature supports care workers including spirituality in care committees to make sense of illness. The questions of death make this needed. Patients need to find love and purpose, and to be accepted as a part of the living universe, but there is no consistent therapy or mechanism/tool to help with this—until VR.

Many patients and families shy away from accepting a chaplain for spiritual healing, especially if they are nondenominational or have no belief in a higher power. But spiritual care is one of the most important proponents of healing in order to find meaning, purpose, wonder, and awe during disease, and during end-of-life in particular. In Chapter 2, we introduced the definition of spirituality as relating to the word "breathe," and that is because it aligns with the Latin word for "spirit," which is linked with breathing and vitality.[2] This alignment was meant to argue that every human has a spiritual need of some sort.

How then do we aid in finding spirituality within this unique medium? Understanding the link between finding meaning, peace, and harmony with the absolute need for a VR therapist role in VR treatment is vital. One begets the other. The process and presence of introduction and prompting from the VR therapist toward the treatment can and will have a profound impact on the possibility for spiritual healing. Every human has spirituality in some unique way. There is something—it can be earthly, divine, or something more deeply personal—that defines the spiritual existence for that person. For some, this is a small piece or less than a piece on which they focus. For others, their spirituality is more meaningful and all-encompassing. Because people tie this so tightly to religions or a denomination, not all people understand or consider themselves spiritual. However, the ability to find meaning *is* spirituality—thus, all who can process and communicate would be considered spiritual. Even a simple mindfulness and reflection practice or experience can define what could be spiritual. Half of America defines spirituality within the realm of religion and refers to the importance in life. Spirituality, unlike religion, is more personal. Care workers cite fear in bringing this up for worry of reaction.[3] Though all humans are spiritual, not all humans have a spiritual life or practice, though beneficence is found in this practice. Practices as simple as nature walks are representative of spirituality.

Another unexpected gain of spiritual life and practice is the feeling of wonder and awe.[4] Being spiritual is finding peace and harmony, unrelated to a god, denomination, church, or similar construct.

Spiritual care provisions align with what it means to humanize death and treat the whole person until that death. Spirituality is the ability to connect with the self. Spirituality takes into consideration how people connect with themselves and with others and find their meaning. Professionals in healthcare do not always align the importance of care with the spiritual need of their patients. Values and beliefs, no matter how they originate, give meaning to spirituality. Spirituality gives light to perspective of purpose in this world. This is a necessary proponent of treatment for the ill and not a natural skill for caregivers.[5]

VR therapy can do more than treat pain and achieve bucket-list goals. It can do more than open the key to the chains holding patients hostage by their ill life. When VR therapy is integrated with a VR therapist and facilitated appropriately, it can unlock meaning and heal the soul. Spiritual care of a patient is about finding what is important to that soul. It is space, personal silence, closure, and conversations about their world. Answering the "why me" or "why now" is key to finding patient's fears and making sense of things.[6] Influencing the work of value-based care, VR therapy heals the whole person.

The Ethics of VR Therapy

Science oftentimes speeds ahead of ethics. Technologies are built and inventions created without enough reflection on how their very existence might negatively affect the common good. This commonplace conundrum is no different when it comes to healthcare and the use of new measures like artificial intelligence (AI). There is no shortage of articles on what the growth of AI might do to the role of the humans. And yet, technology and science continue the creation and advancement of this awesome capability. VR is not exempted from this trend. Currently, if VR is not acknowledged as a treatment modality, then informed consent is not obtained. All interventions, including VR, should be treated with the same protocol as other procedures. Thus, the use of VR should not be viewed as less than or extra. It is a serious treatment with absolute demand for consent, process, flow, and facilitation.

Process and the Development of Best Practices
Onboarding
Most patients are new to virtual-reality therapy, so it is important to gain their trust and confidence at the beginning of a session. Overwhelmed with tests, pharmacies, multiple appointments and dealing with symptoms, patients in palliative care oftentimes have resistance to trying something new. This can be overcome simply by the palliative-care doctor recommending VR to their patients for pain management and anxiety relief. The admissions administrator can also be instrumental in recommending VR to patients upon check in. The simple addition of wearing a white lab coat can reassure patients that they are receiving professional treatment.

With hospice patients, it's important to access their receptivity to trying VR. Some are quite responsive and it's a welcome break in the monotony of being bed-bound and watching daytime television. If a patient is sleeping, do not disturb them.

Many patients view VR as technology that is for gaming only and something they might have seen their grandchildren or children playing. Although play and fun are strong elements in immersive experiences, it is important to meet patients where they are.

Onboarding is a time to discuss with new patients their pain levels, anxiety levels, and any fears such as claustrophobia, underwater phobias, vertigo, and so forth. Reading a patient correctly can be the key to a successful immersive therapy session. It is also crucial to explain what VR is, how it can help them, and letting them know that at any time, they can remove the headset. Giving patients, when appropriate, a choice is also seminal in creating a positive session. A menu of curated VR could include experiences to:

- ◆ Enhance quality of life: travel, adventure, fun, inspiring, and playful.
- ◆ Relieve and reduce pain: engaging, stimulating, interactive, all-encompassing.
- ◆ Alleviate anxiety and fear: calming, meditative, beautiful nature, awe inspiring.
- ◆ Provide emotional and spiritual support: meditative, awe inspiring.

In end-of-life care, many patients are seeking some form of spiritual solace. Patients will ask to go to church, hear gospel music, visit Jerusalem, the Wailing Wall and many other awe-inspiring sites. Carefully curating experiences that touch the soul can provide an inspiring and transformative moment for these patients.

Session

Fitting the headset comfortably on the patient and making sure that they are seated in a relaxed position is essential. Eliminate all distraction from phones (turn the ringer off), outside conversations, and noise, if possible. If this is a home-care visit, gently encourage other family members to be quiet or leave the room and close the door. Loading multiple experiences—for example, a skydiving experience, an underwater adventure, or space travel, or multiple experiences of the same VR episodes—onto a headset is another strategy for ensuring continuous deep immersion. Being sensitive and present to a patient enables one to curate the session in real time. One can tell from body language how a patient is responding and if there is a need to change out the content. Casting the VR to an iPad will enable the immersive therapist to help patients with interactivity and get them used to navigating in virtual space.

It is helpful to start a session with a pleasant and entertaining experience such as immersive music, art, or even a Broadway performance. It is immediately arresting and puts the patient at ease. Underwater experiences that transport patients to another world are also calming and immediate mood enhancers. With the initial novelty of being in a completely 360-degree environment, patients oftentimes want more content, more engagement, and longer sessions.

Post Session

Taking the time for reflection after the experience is essential because it gives patients a voice. Many patients long to be heard and often describe feelings that lie buried underneath the hurried schedule of visits with professionals dispensing medication and the charting of the day-to-day conditions. Cultivating good communication and good listening skills as well as patience and compassion greatly benefit immersive sessions. VR can lead patients into contemplation, meditation, and self-transcendent experiences (STEs), so the dialogue after a session can be very meaningful. The VR therapist can have multiple roles: facilitator, coach, guide, shaman, and healer.

Finding out what was engaging, what experiences they'd like to repeat, and what a patient would like to further explore will lead to future successful immersive therapy sessions. What were their key takeaways? Did an experience resonate with a patient, change their mood, and cause a shift in their awareness? Oftentimes, VR can be a break in the routine of illness and an opportunity for awe.

Fieldwork: Meeting Patients Where They Are

Miss Dorothy was a patient with pancreatic cancer. She was extremely fatigued, confused, and had little interest in her surroundings the day of her appointment at the palliative-care clinic. Prior to her session, her blood pressure was exceedingly low. Based on her low energy level, during her first time with VR, she was shown energizing and life-enhancing content, such as travel and physical activity. She came to life during a VR experience of surfing in Tahiti. Suddenly, she was on her feet with her arms extended, walking the tip of an imaginary surfboard. Her body language showed her ducking sprays of whitewater and riding huge waves. She was extremely exuberant and animated in her response to VR therapy. When her blood pressure was measured again at the end of her session, it was normal, and she insisted on going shopping and driving the car—something she hadn't done in a number of months. Miss Dorothy wanted to take the VR headset home.

Sometimes inducing awe is not a panacea for a patient. Sometimes anger and rage about the diagnosis supersedes all. Such was the case of a thirty-five-year-old obstetrician/gynecologist who battled breast cancer. Dr. Jennifer had delivered thousands of babies and was a breast cancer survivor. However, when she went for an annual checkup to determine if she could have her own baby, she found out that her cancer had metastasized, and her body was riddled with malignant growths. She entered palliative care as a stage-4 patient and VR was recommended for her pain and depression. Her first session was transformational; she was energized, exuberant, and danced around her living room. She was all-in to use immersive therapy. Her husband, delighted at her response, purchased a headset for home use.

During the next sessions, she exhibited increasing anger. She couldn't let go of her guilt, shame, and defeat at the recurrence of her diagnosis. Her rational, analytical mind prevented her from moving forward with VR therapy. She was provided multiple published studies on the positive effects of VR for pain management and quality of life. As her aggressive cancer progressed, she grew more resistant. In a number of weeks, she entered hospice care and died shortly thereafter.

VR therapy is also beneficial to family members and caregivers. Nancy's infant was born critically ill with birth defects and was admitted to hospice. Additionally, she had a three-year precocious son, Tony. In the face of the ensuing tragedy that the infant could not sustain life, VR therapy brought solace and comfort to both mom and her son. When Tony experienced VR, Nancy found grace in the pleasure of just watching her son be a child again in the midst of so much grown-up stress. After experiencing meditative VR, she exclaimed, "When you're in such a difficult point in your life, it's really helpful to have that kind of support. I'm very thankful… It feels calming. It's probably the most calming moment I've had in a very long, long time."

Technical Skills

The rapid evolution and emergence of VR as a successful and exciting new method of therapy for the seriously ill has been astounding in the last decade. A growing number of medical, health, and wellness professionals have been drawn to this new field of research and practice. Working with VR does require that a VR therapist have some basic skills with VR technology so that they are comfortable with virtual-reality software and hardware. These technical skills can be easily learned, particularly when a new VR therapist is excited about working with VR.

VR therapists need to be able to download and access the VR "content," the virtual-reality experiences that are being used with the patients. The VR experiences come from numerous sources, including subscription series, YouTube 360 videos, and VR platforms like the Meta Quest store and Steam. Unless a VR headset comes preloaded with VR content, VR experiences need to be downloaded to the chosen headset.

VR therapists also need to have basic skills with the VR headsets that are used. VR HMDs are constantly being upgraded and improved. Meta, Apple, HTC Vive, Pico, and more are being used in hospitals, health, and wellness facilities around the world. At the same time, the use of VR headsets has grown exponentially in education, gaming, design, many industries, and consumers in general. Headsets have become more popular, ubiquitous, and accessible.

Along with skills in downloading programs, VR therapists need to learn to practice good VR maintenance. The headsets need to be cleaned and sterilized after each use. This process requires the use of sterilizing wipes or the use of an ultraviolet-C light-emitting diode (UVC LED) decontamination system such as a Cleanbox, which sterilizes the headset in a few minutes.

Similar to a mobile phone or personal computer's operating system, the headset operating system receives updates that need attention. For example, Meta pushes out updates and optimizes the applications periodically and the VR therapist needs to stay current and be ready to troubleshoot the systems.

Important to many health facilities is the tracking of data and patient progress. VR sessions are often combined with the collection of internal review board (IRB) data that is used in ongoing research or studies. The simple tracking of pain levels, anxiety, blood pressure, and heart rate before and after VR sessions is useful for monitoring the well-being of patients and to track the success of a VR therapy session.

Traditionally, hospitals use the Wong-Baker FACES Pain Rating Scale to measure pain, as shown in Figure 9.1.

Some VR headsets, such as the HP Reverb G2 Omnicept, can collect data internally, including biometrics, eye tracking, engagement, breath rate, heart rate, and so forth. By collecting and analyzing data using AI, certain diagnoses can be predicted earlier and a customized treatment program developed.

Varjo, Pico, Neo, and Vive are HMDs that have eye-tracking capabilities that enable interactivity and customization of user-specific features in VR. For a patient with limited mobility or cognitive skills, this can be crucial in providing a positive and uniquely tailored VR experience.

Immersive technology's capability is advancing exponentially with AI and has the potential to take medical and well-being applications to the next level. Cutting-edge VR technology is being employed by teams of medical researchers worldwide who are working with a wide range of topics that have the potential

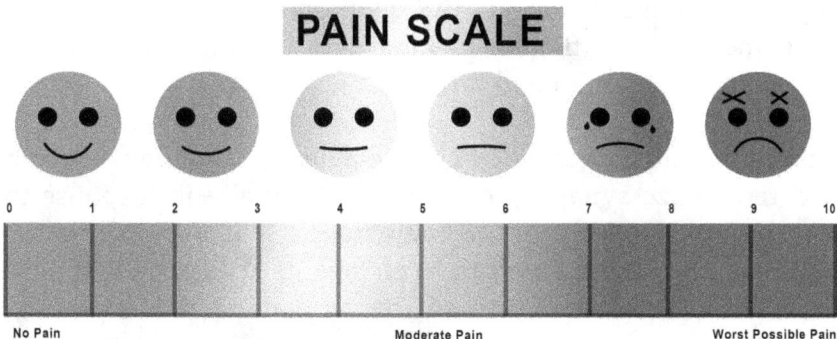

PAIN SCALE

| 0 | 1 | 2 | 3 | 4 | 5 | 6 | 7 | 8 | 9 | 10 |

No Pain   Moderate Pain   Worst Possible Pain

FIGURE 9.1

to revolutionize medicine. One team in Rotterdam is using AI to interpret magnetic resonance imaging (MRI) and computed tomography (CT) data to build 3D extrusions of patient thoracic cavities. The immersive 3D extrusions are loaded into VR so that surgeons can have pre-operative planning and visualization prior to procedures.[7]

The Future of Virtual Therapy

Neuroplasticity and VR

Neurologists are using VR to research neuroplasticity and the brain's ability to heal and rehabilitate the body.

> It's happening at Georgia Institute of Technology, where Nick Housley runs the Sensorimotor Integration Lab. There, patients undergoing neurorehabilitation, including those recovering from a stroke, are outfitted with robotic devices called Motus, which are strapped to their arms and legs. The goal: to speed up recovery and assist with rehabilitation exercises. Patients and practitioners using the system wear virtual-reality headsets. The Motus device sends feedback to the clinician, who can guide the patient through exercises designed to recover movements they have lost. "The headset tells you really critical things, like how much force someone's muscle can put out," Housley says. "It can also tailor an intervention—for example, if someone has difficulty picking up a cup of coffee, you can guide them in real time."[8]

Neuroplasticity is described as "the ability of the brain to form and reorganize synaptic connections, especially in response to learning or experience or following injury."[9] "It is defined as the ability of the nervous system to change its activity in response to intrinsic or extrinsic stimuli by reorganizing its structure, functions, or connections after injuries, such as a stroke or traumatic brain injury."[10]

Much has been published on VR's ability to rewire the brain. One well-known study, The Walk Again project, uses VR therapy to help rewire the cognitive connection between the brain and the spinal cord. The Walk Again project was developed at Duke University by neurophysiologists Miguel Nicolelis and John Chapin. Over years of research with brain-machine interface (BMI) and robotic exoskeletons, they developed highly effective VR interfaces that allowed the patients to visualize their limbs and practice movement. Patients were put in exoskeleton suits to manipulate paralyzed limbs and at the same time were shown VR simulations of their own feet moving normally. The idea was to stimulate new neural pathways by tricking and stimulating the brain. The therapy has been successful with some patients regaining feeling, regaining bladder control and control of paralyzed legs. The research now goes on worldwide and with newer VR systems that allow for more patient access to time spent in rehabilitation. Nicolelis predicts that the therapy will extend beyond spinal cord injuries to "stroke victims and other neurological disorders."[11]

MindMaze is a company that is taking immersive technology far into the future. It was founded by Tej Tadi, who has been a pioneer and a world leader in using VR in immersive physical and neurological therapies. Since 2012, he has combined VR, AR, MR, biosensors, AI, haptic interfaces, facial recognition, smart peripherals, and the latest advances in immersive, interactive neuroscience. He has led groundbreaking research into new approaches to neurorehabilitation, enhanced recovery, learning, memory, pain, sports, and more. His goal is to improve brain health universally and to bring advances in neuroscience to everyday life (https://www.mindmaze.com).

The VR Pharmacy

Brennan Spiegel, director of health-services research at Cedars-Sinai Medical Center, directs the Center for Outcomes Research and Education, which maintains one of the largest and most widely cited therapeutic virtual-reality programs in the world. He has led countless research projects exploring numerous aspects of virtual medicine, and one of his goals for the future has always been the development of a VR pharmacy. He envisions a future apothecary of immersive experiences that can be carefully curated and prescribed by immersive therapists. In his book *VRx: How Virtual Medicine will Revolutionize Medicine*, Spiegel wrote, "If VR is a therapy, then we need a VR pharmacy. As a doctor, I need shelves full of VR treatments that are safe, effective, and that I can personalize for each individual patient."[12] "When used in the right way, in the right people, and at the right time, VR brings wonder and beauty to mankind. If nothing else, it offers joy. And joy is good. We should leverage that."[13]

The archive of VR therapeutic content is growing rapidly. Numerous experiences have been created by medical and creative teams that have achieved FDA approval. The list includes AppliedVR, MindMaze, Eye-Sync, SNAP + SyncAR, Penumbra, and others. More and more content developers are creating VR for medical and therapeutic work. It is an exciting time to stay tuned in to this emerging body of work and an exhilarating challenge to stay current with the latest advances in VR technology.

With the growth of immersive VR and XR medicine, programs in hospitals and the health and wellness industries, the training in medical schools, research institutes and universities worldwide, the future is immersive.

References

1 Scribbr. (2023, November). 77% of healthcare organizations surveyed have implemented virtual reality (VR) to support medical training – or are planning to; what are some of the use cases? Retrieved from https://www.medtechdive.com/press-release/20231 120-77-of-healthcare-organizations-surveyed-have-implemented-virtual-reality/#:~:text=from%20your%20inbox.-,77%25%20 of%20Healthcare%20Organizations%20Surveyed%20Have%20 Implemented%20Virtual%20Reality%20(VR,Some%20of%20 the%20Use%20Cases%3F

2 García-Navarro, E.B., Medina-Ortega, A., & García Navarro, S. (2021). Spirituality in patients at the end of life—Is it necessary? A qualitative

approach to the protagonists. *International Journal of Environmental Research and Public Health*, *19*(1), 227.

3   Hopeck, P. (2020). Spiritual reassurance: Experiences of care workers during end of life. *Journal of Communication & Religion*, *43*(4), 77–91.

4   DeFord, B. (2023). The personal and the professional: Mindfulness, spiritual life and health care [article under review]. The spiritual cycle of providing professional health care. *OBM Integrated and Complementary Medicine*, *8*(1).

5   García-Navarro, E.B., Medina-Ortega, A., & García Navarro, S. (2021). Spirituality in patients at the end of life—is it necessary? A qualitative approach to the protagonists. *International Journal of Environmental Research and Public Health*, *19*(1), 227.

6   Batstone, E., Bailey, C., & Hallett, N. (2020). Spiritual care provision to end-of-life patients: A systematic literature review. *Journal of Clinical Nursing*, *29*(19–20), 3609–3624.

7   Sadeghi, A., Maat, W.P.W.M., Taverne, Y.J.H.J., Cornelissen, R., Dingemans, A-M.C., Bogers, J.J.C., & Mahtab, E.A. (2021, March 16). Virtual reality and artificial intelligence for 3-dimensional planning of lung segmentectomies. *JTCVS Techniques, 7*, 309–321. https://doi/10.1016/j.xjtc.2021.03.016

8   Brodsky, S. (2022, March 4). How virtual reality is expanding health care. *Time*. Retrieved from https://time.com/6155085/virtual-reality-improve-health-care/

9   Oxford English Dictionary. (n.d.). "Neuroplasticity." Retrieved from https://www.oed.com

10 Puderbaugh, M., & Emmady, P.D. (2023, May 1). Neuroplasticity. National institutes of health, National center for biotechnology information. Retrieved from https://www.ncbi.nlm.nih.gov/books/NBK557811/#:~:text=It%20is%20defined%20as%20the, traumatic%20brain%20injury%20(TBI)

11 Stone, M. (2023, October 3). How VR is helping paraplegics walk again. *Forbes*. Retrieved from https://www.forbes.com/sites/delltechnologies/2018/01/16/how-vr-is-helping-paraplegics-walk-again/?sh=575ce35275d0

12 Spiegel, B. (2020). *VRx: How virtual therapeutics will revolutionize medicine*. New York: Basic Books, p. 188.

13 Spiegel, B. (2020). *VRx: How virtual therapeutics will revolutionize medicine*. New York: Basic Books, p. 247.

Index

Note: **Bold** page numbers refer to tables and *italic* page numbers refer to figures.

For Product Safety Concerns and Information please contact our EU
representative GPSR@taylorandfrancis.com
Taylor & Francis Verlag GmbH, Kaufingerstraße 24, 80331 München, Germany